Colon Cancer Survivors Coloring & Activity Book

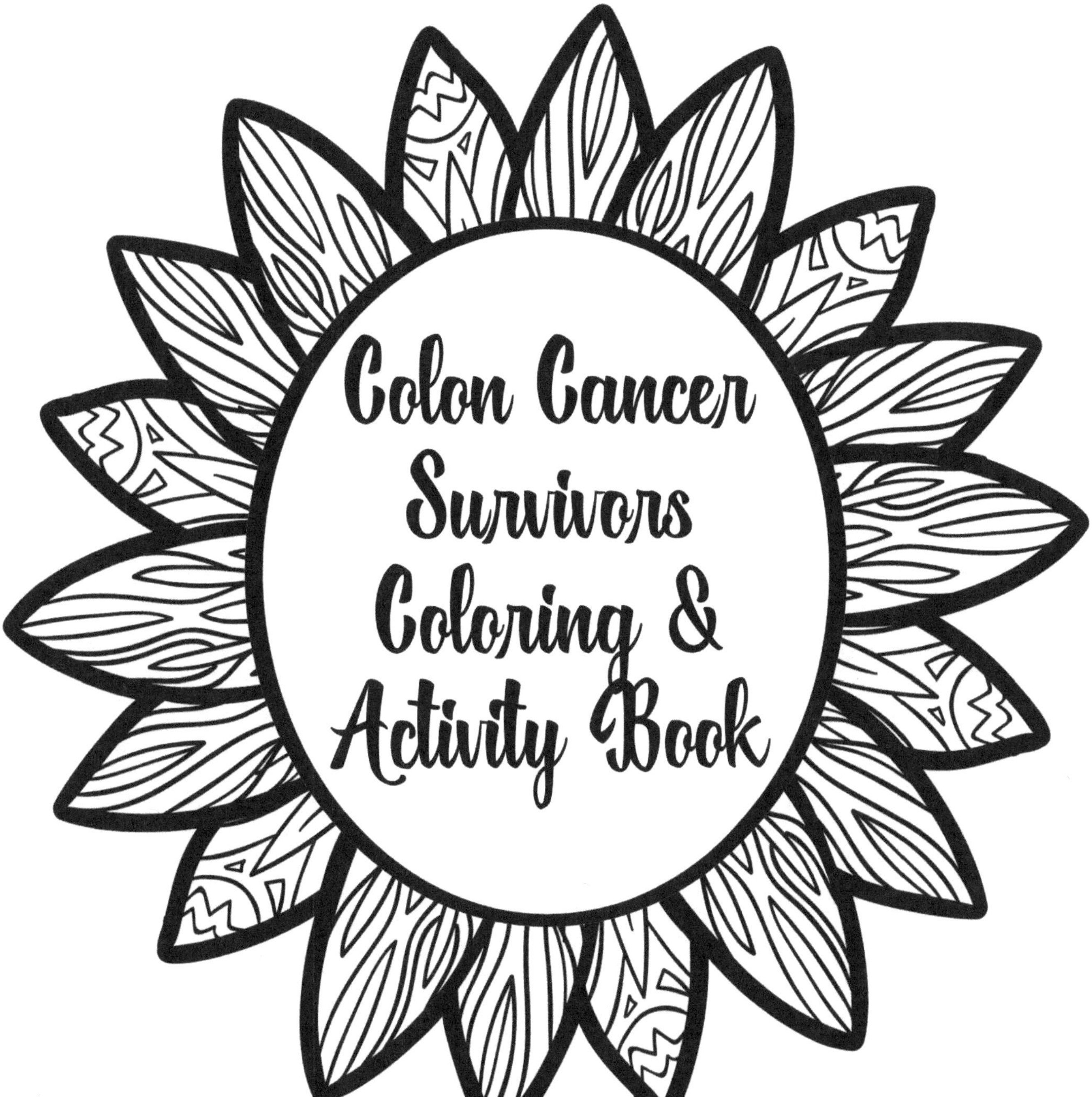

This extraordinary stress-relieving, relaxing coloring, and activity book were particularly designed for all Colorectal Cancer Survivors. Experience hours of calming pencil coloring and an entertaining assortment of activity sheets. Also included are journaling pages to record your moods and emotions and feel inspired by inspirational quotes.

Pass the time while you recuperate, by indulging yourself in joyful and brilliant coloring, believing in yourself, but best of all, self-care!

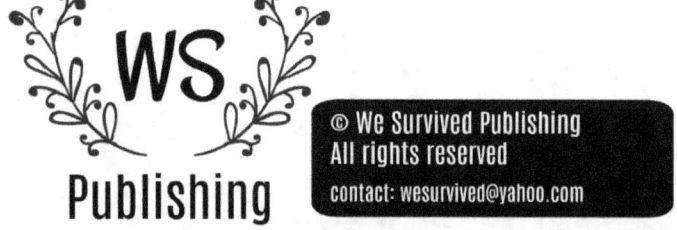

THE OSTOMY BAG (POUCH)

Living with an ostomy bag (pouch) is an enormous adjustment in lifestyle, and for a good number of people, it's incredibly exasperating, challenging, and difficult to adjust.

Some patients were diagnosed with colon, bowel, or rectal cancer or other illnesses, preparing themselves for an upcoming colostomy or ileostomy surgery necessitating an ostomy appliance, while others underwent emergency surgery, thus waking up revealing a bag connected to their abdomen. (After healing, a reversal or "takedown" is possible).

Hopefully, post surgery patients learn how to properly care for their ostomies before they return home and ultimately adapt to this unfamiliar system. But, not all people are as well educated by healthcare workers and return home feeling perplexed, disappointed, and helpless.

How Are You Feeling Today?

MENTAL HEALTH **PHYSICAL HEALTH**

positive	exhausted	healthy	ill
great	helpless	active	in pain
accomplished	hopeless	energetic	weight gain
frustrated	guilty	fatigued	weight loss
isolated	bothersome	hungry	thirsty
depressed	loveless	no appetite	nauseous
discouraged	ugly	insomnia	bloated
lonely	bored	achy	blockage

Notes: _____

_____

_____

_____

_____

_____

_____

_____

_____

_____

_____

_____

_____

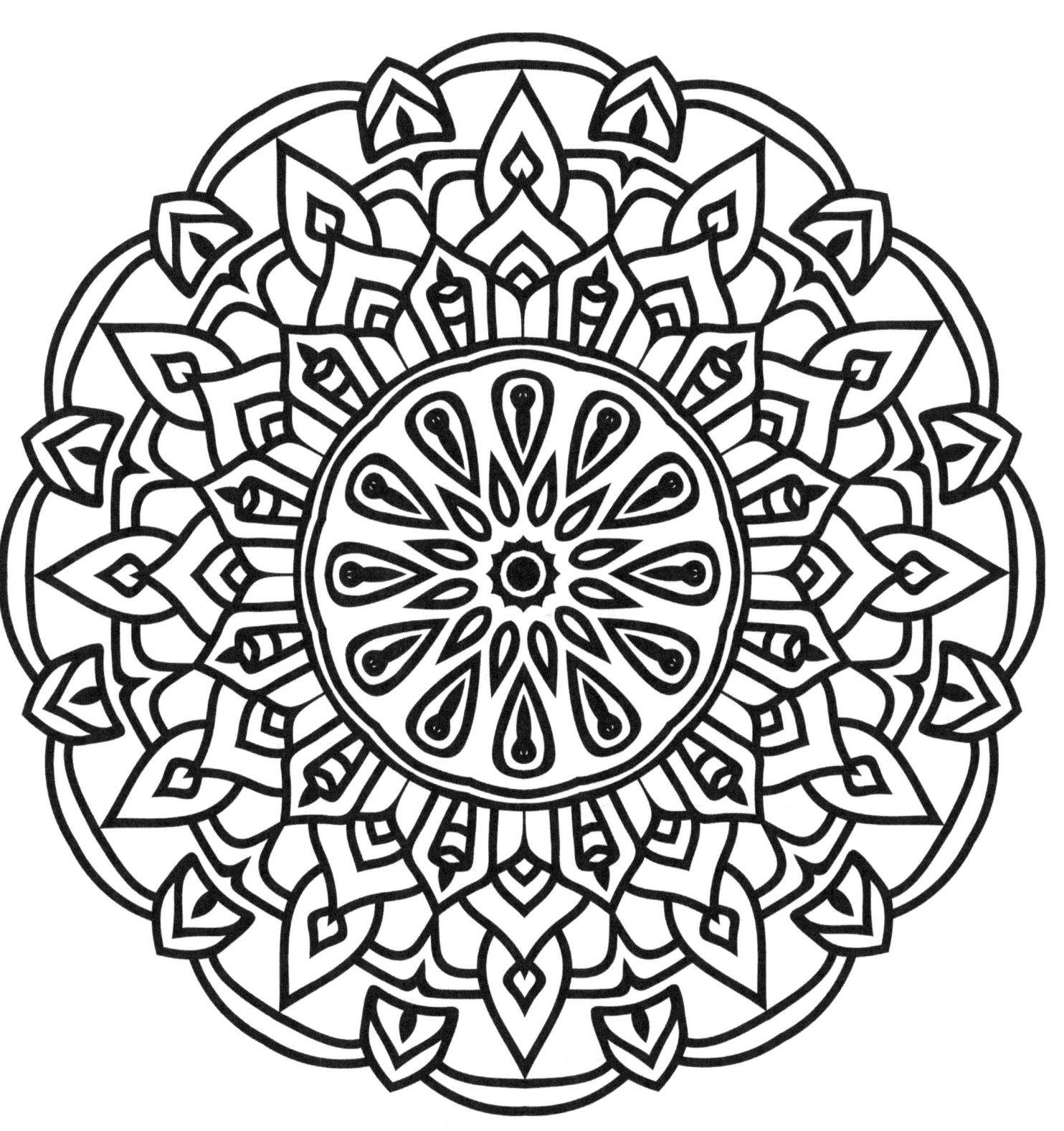

How Are You Feeling Today?

MENTAL HEALTH **PHYSICAL HEALTH**

	positive		exhausted		healthy		ill
	great		helpless		active		in pain
	accomplished		hopeless		energetic		weight gain
	frustrated		guilty		fatigued		weight loss
	isolated		bothersome		hungry		thirsty
	depressed		loveless		no appetite		nauseous
	discouraged		ugly		insomnia		bloated
	lonely		bored		achy		blockage

Notes: _____

_____

_____

_____

_____

_____

_____

_____

_____

_____

_____

_____

_____

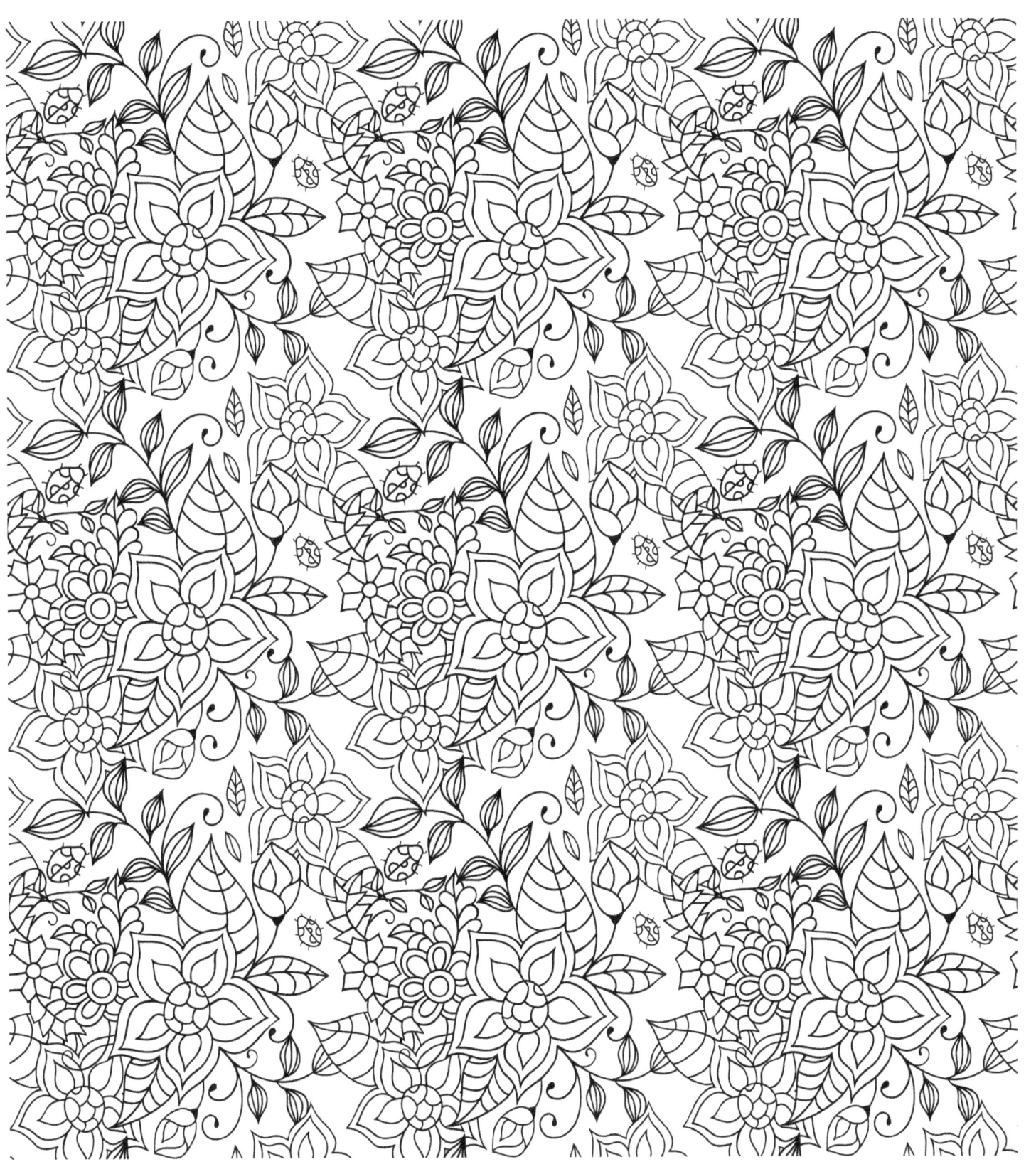

How Are You Feeling Today?

MENTAL HEALTH   **PHYSICAL HEALTH**

positive	exhausted	healthy	ill
great	helpless	active	in pain
accomplished	hopeless	energetic	weight gain
frustrated	guilty	fatigued	weight loss
isolated	bothersome	hungry	thirsty
depressed	loveless	no appetite	nauseous
discouraged	ugly	insomnia	bloated
lonely	bored	achy	blockage

Notes: _____

_____

_____

_____

_____

_____

_____

_____

_____

_____

_____

_____

_____

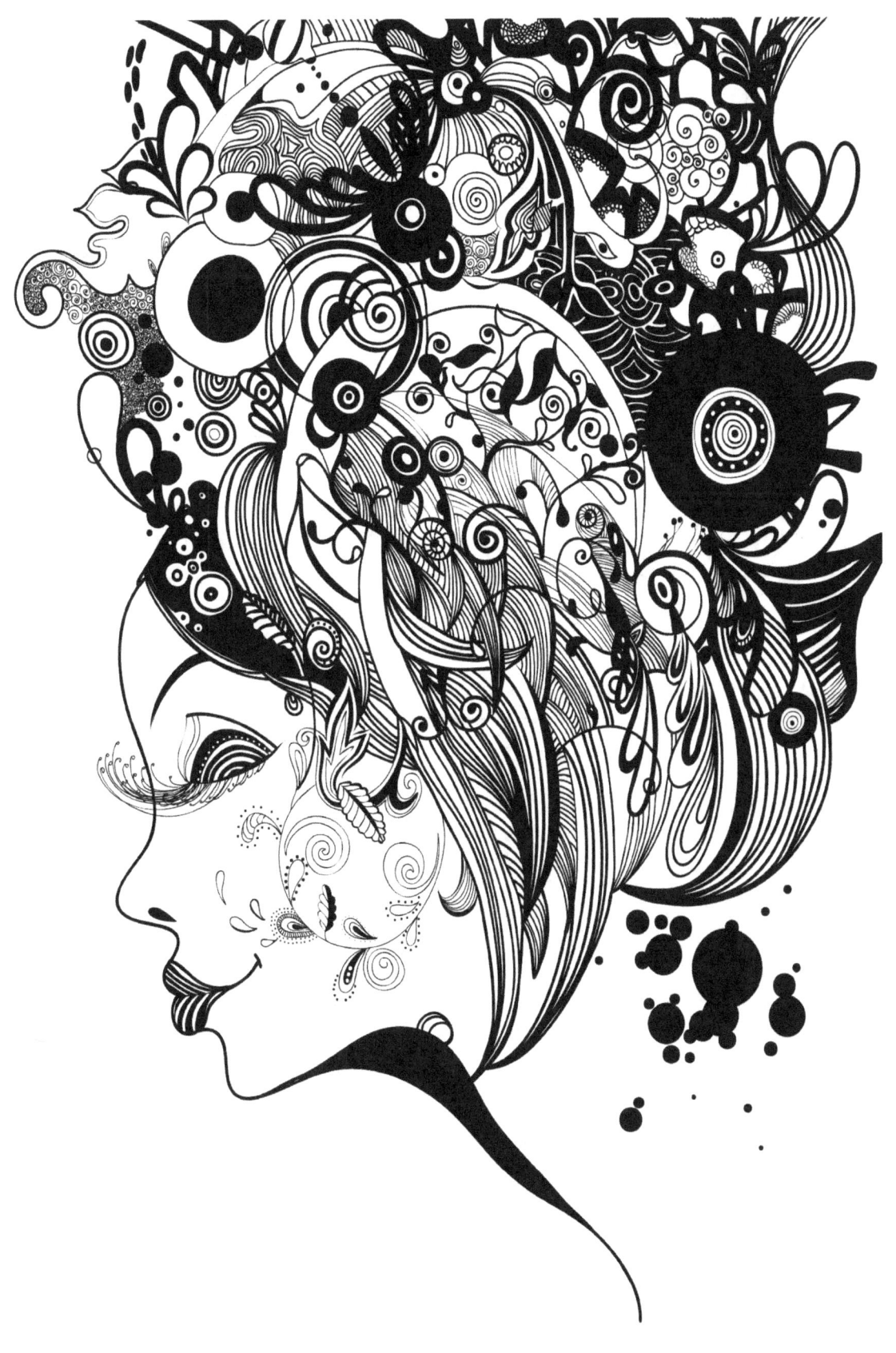

How Are You Feeling Today?

MENTAL HEALTH ; **PHYSICAL HEALTH**

positive	exhausted	healthy	ill
great	helpless	active	in pain
accomplished	hopeless	energetic	weight gain
frustrated	guilty	fatigued	weight loss
isolated	bothersome	hungry	thirsty
depressed	loveless	no appetite	nauseous
discouraged	ugly	insomnia	bloated
lonely	bored	achy	blockage

Notes: _____

_____

_____

_____

_____

_____

_____

_____

_____

_____

_____

_____

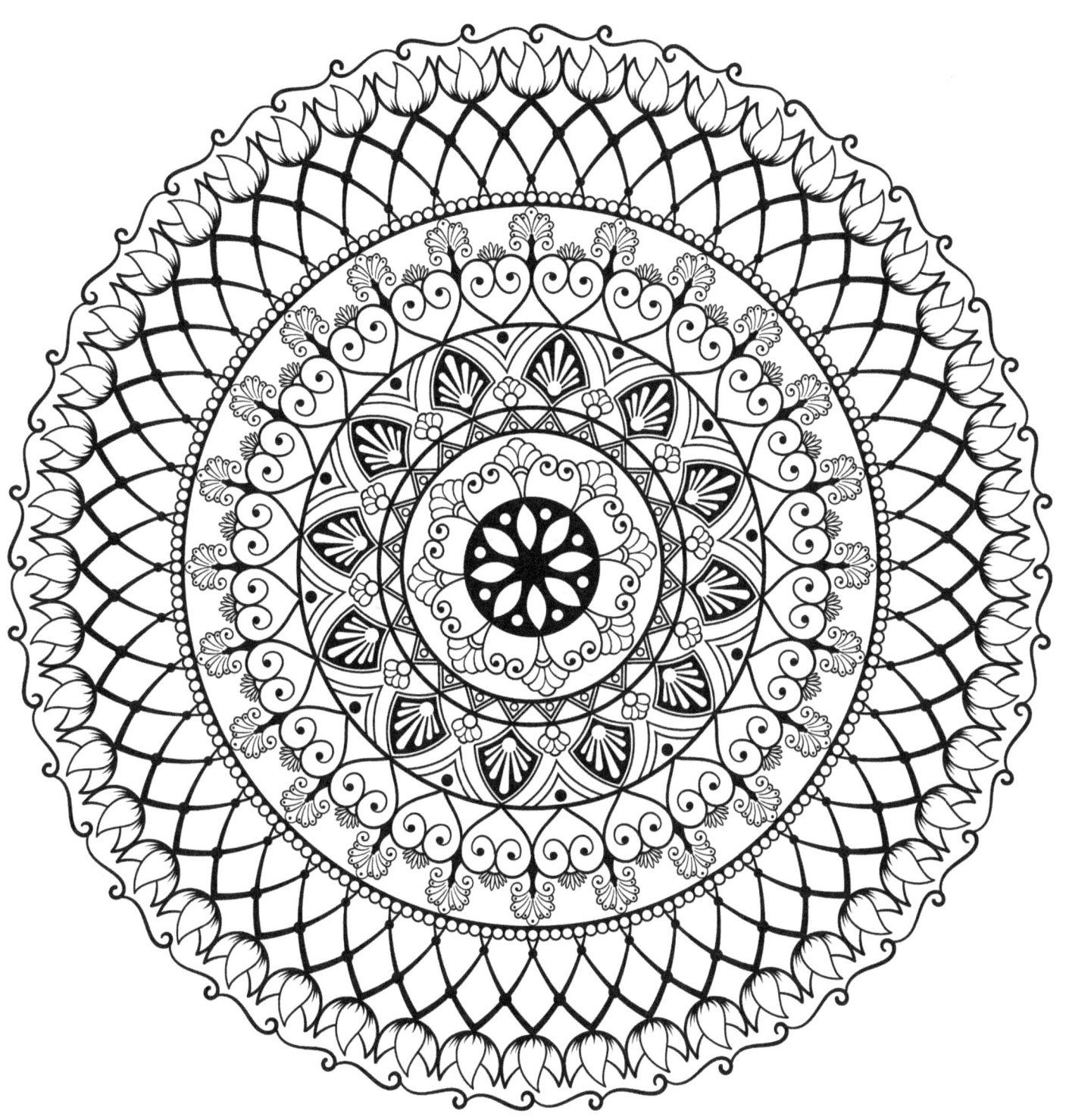

How Are You Feeling Today?

MENTAL HEALTH　　　　　　　　**PHYSICAL HEALTH**

positive	exhausted	healthy	ill
great	helpless	active	in pain
accomplished	hopeless	energetic	weight gain
frustrated	guilty	fatigued	weight loss
isolated	bothersome	hungry	thirsty
depressed	loveless	no appetite	nauseous
discouraged	ugly	insomnia	bloated
lonely	bored	achy	blockage

Notes: _____

_____

_____

_____

_____

_____

_____

_____

_____

_____

_____

_____

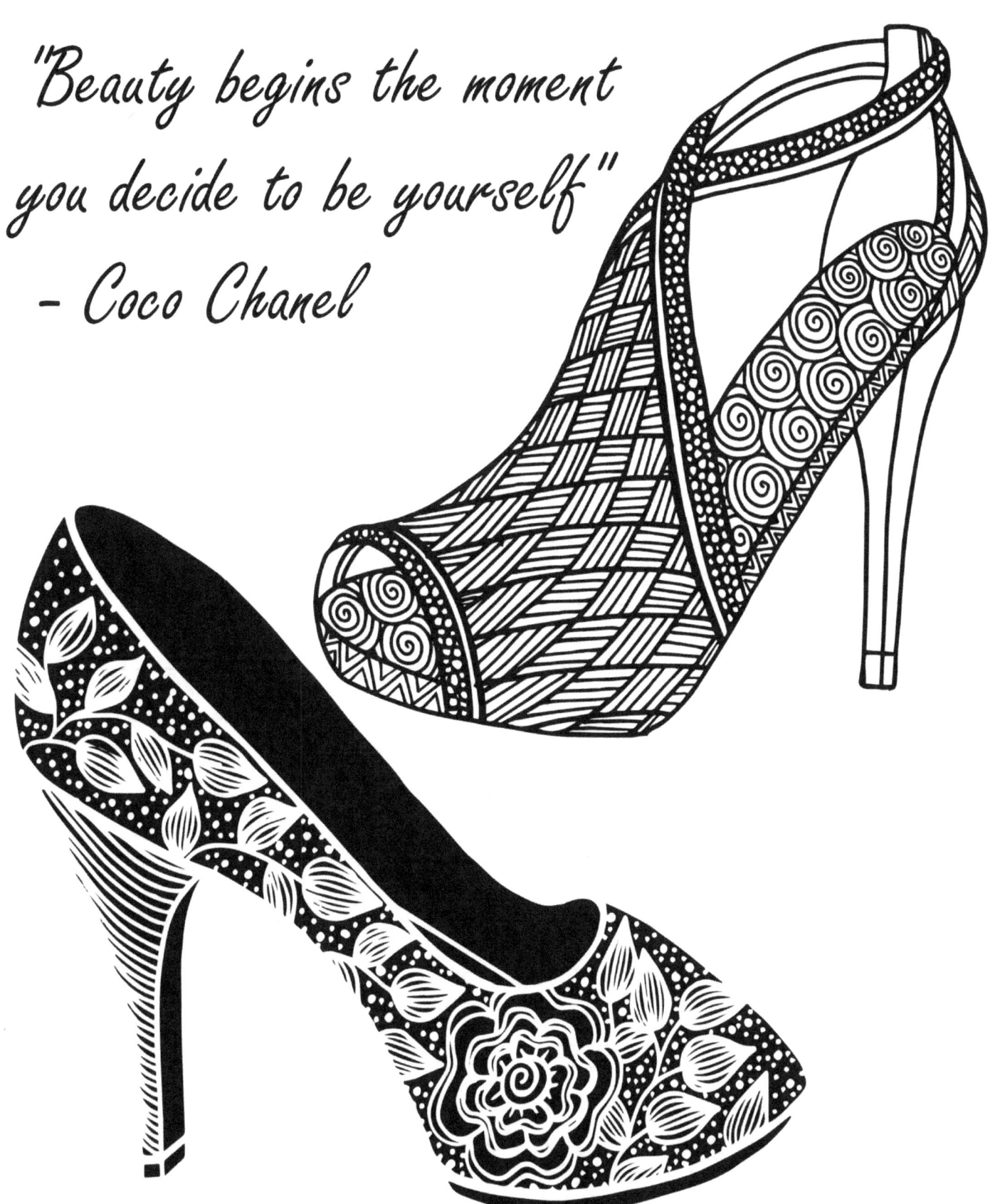

How Are You Feeling Today?

MENTAL HEALTH   **PHYSICAL HEALTH**

positive	exhausted	healthy	ill
great	helpless	active	in pain
accomplished	hopeless	energetic	weight gain
frustrated	guilty	fatigued	weight loss
isolated	bothersome	hungry	thirsty
depressed	loveless	no appetite	nauseous
discouraged	ugly	insomnia	bloated
lonely	bored	achy	blockage

Notes: _____

_____

_____

_____

_____

_____

_____

_____

_____

_____

_____

_____

_____

How Are You Feeling Today?

MENTAL HEALTH **PHYSICAL HEALTH**

positive	exhausted	healthy	ill
great	helpless	active	in pain
accomplished	hopeless	energetic	weight gain
frustrated	guilty	fatigued	weight loss
isolated	bothersome	hungry	thirsty
depressed	loveless	no appetite	nauseous
discouraged	ugly	insomnia	bloated
lonely	bored	achy	blockage

Notes: _____

_____

_____

_____

_____

_____

_____

_____

_____

_____

_____

_____

_____

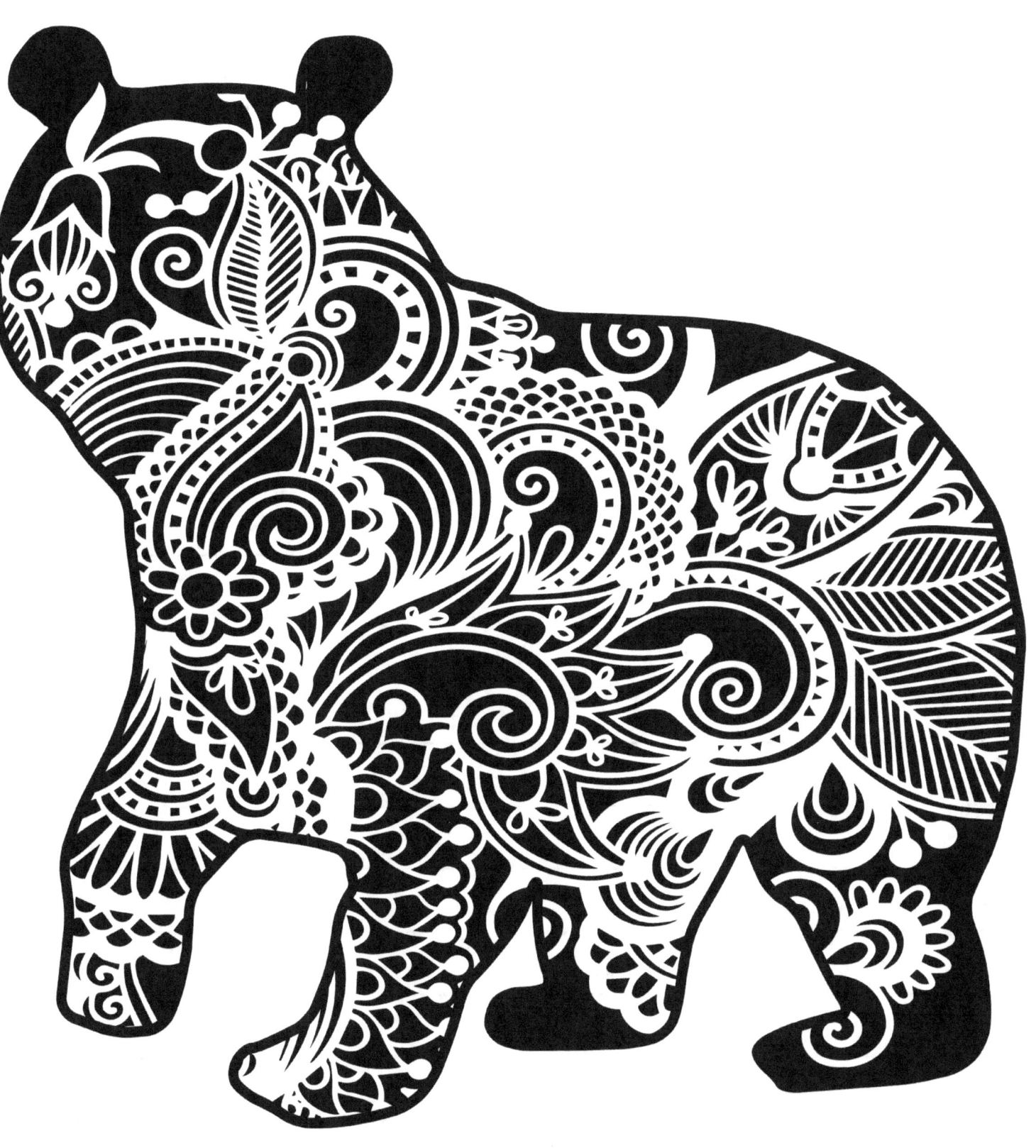

How Are You Feeling Today?

MENTAL HEALTH **PHYSICAL HEALTH**

positive	exhausted	healthy	ill
great	helpless	active	in pain
accomplished	hopeless	energetic	weight gain
frustrated	guilty	fatigued	weight loss
isolated	bothersome	hungry	thirsty
depressed	loveless	no appetite	nauseous
discouraged	ugly	insomnia	bloated
lonely	bored	achy	blockage

Notes: _____

_____

_____

_____

_____

_____

_____

_____

_____

_____

_____

_____

_____

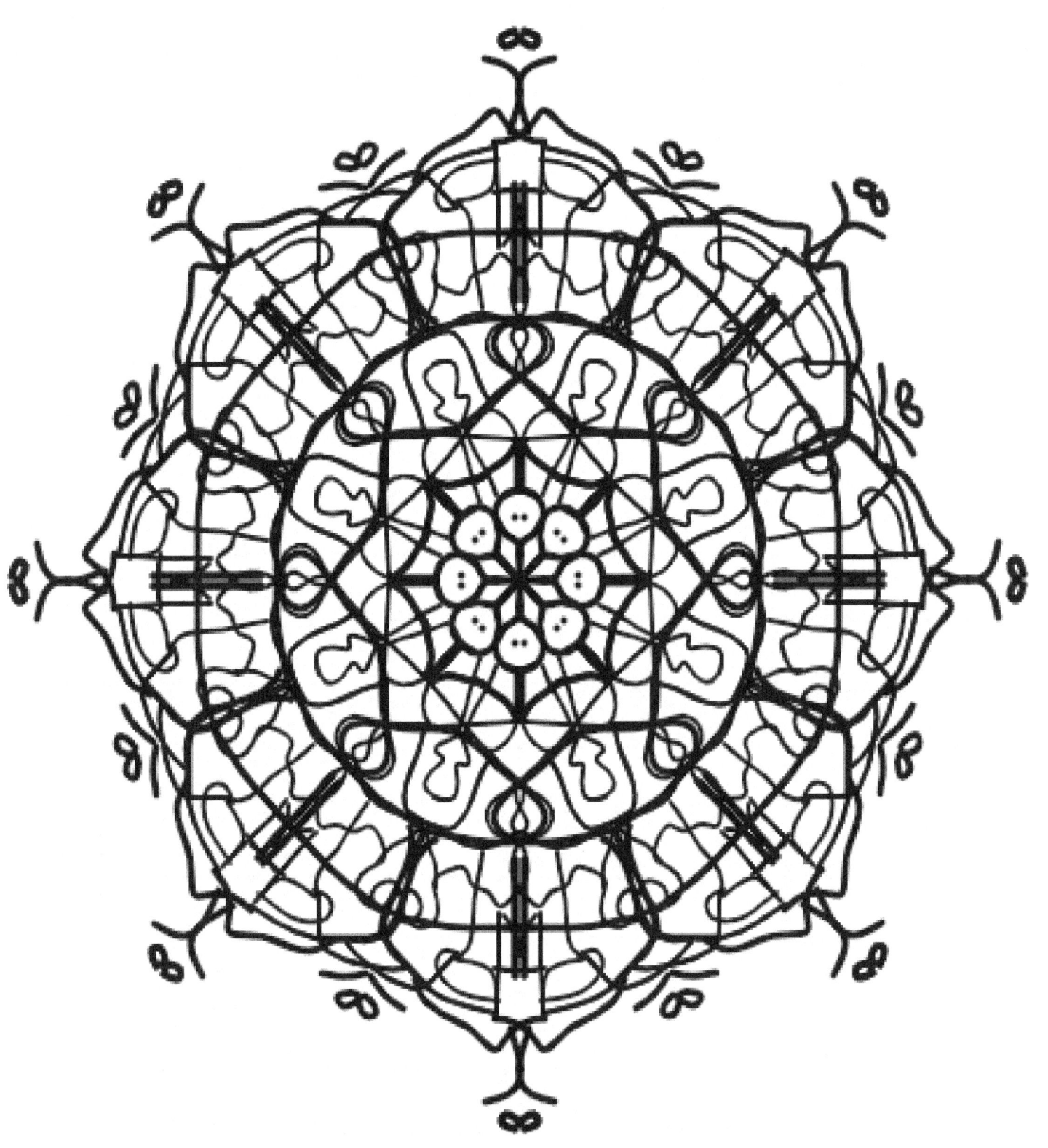

How Are You Feeling Today?

MENTAL HEALTH   **PHYSICAL HEALTH**

positive	exhausted	healthy	ill
great	helpless	active	in pain
accomplished	hopeless	energetic	weight gain
frustrated	guilty	fatigued	weight loss
isolated	bothersome	hungry	thirsty
depressed	loveless	no appetite	nauseous
discouraged	ugly	insomnia	bloated
lonely	bored	achy	blockage

Notes: _____

_____

_____

_____

_____

_____

_____

_____

_____

_____

_____

_____

_____

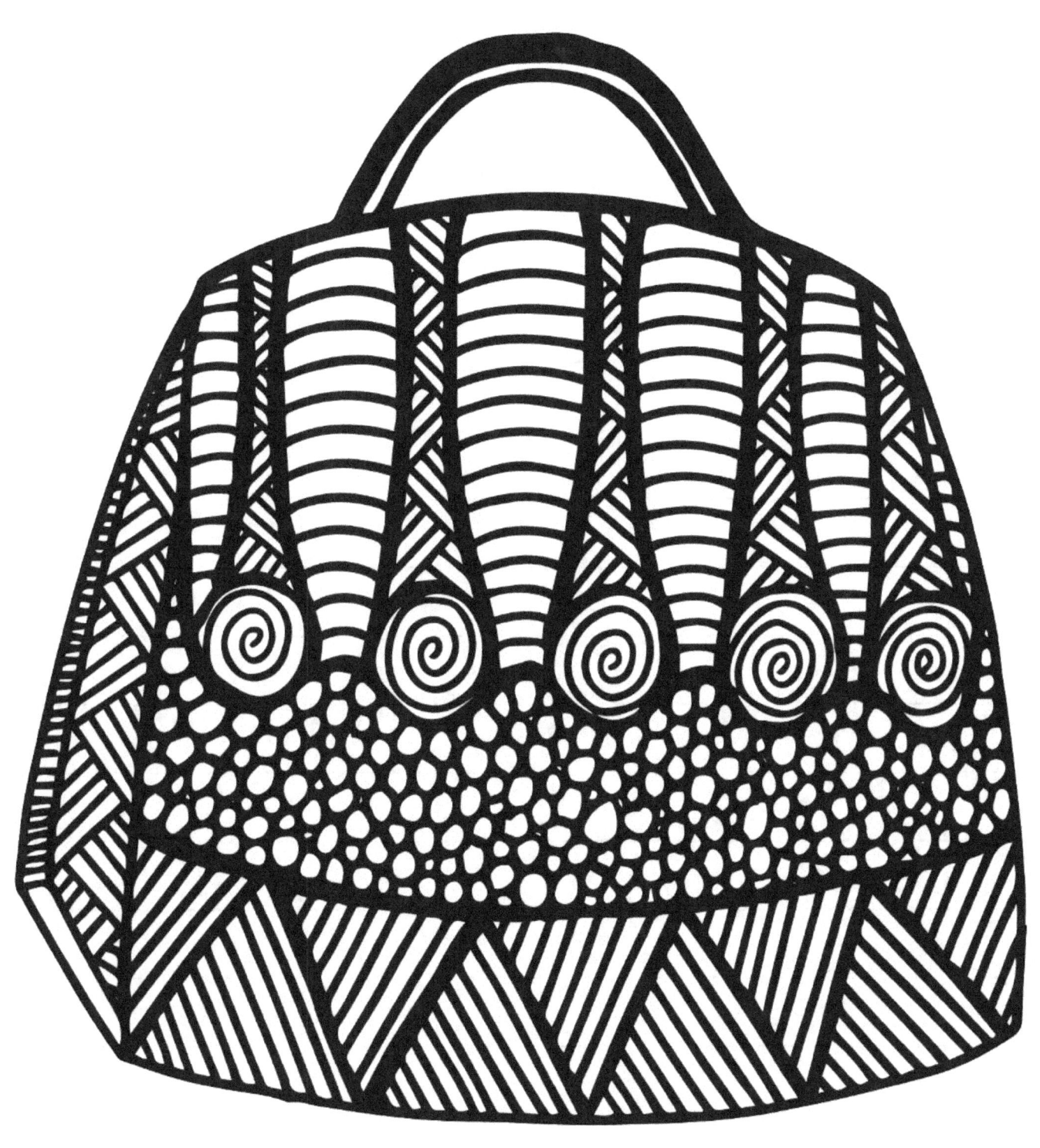

How Are You Feeling Today?

MENTAL HEALTH   **PHYSICAL HEALTH**

positive	exhausted	healthy	ill
great	helpless	active	in pain
accomplished	hopeless	energetic	weight gain
frustrated	guilty	fatigued	weight loss
isolated	bothersome	hungry	thirsty
depressed	loveless	no appetite	nauseous
discouraged	ugly	insomnia	bloated
lonely	bored	achy	blockage

Notes: _____

_____

_____

_____

_____

_____

_____

_____

_____

_____

_____

_____

_____

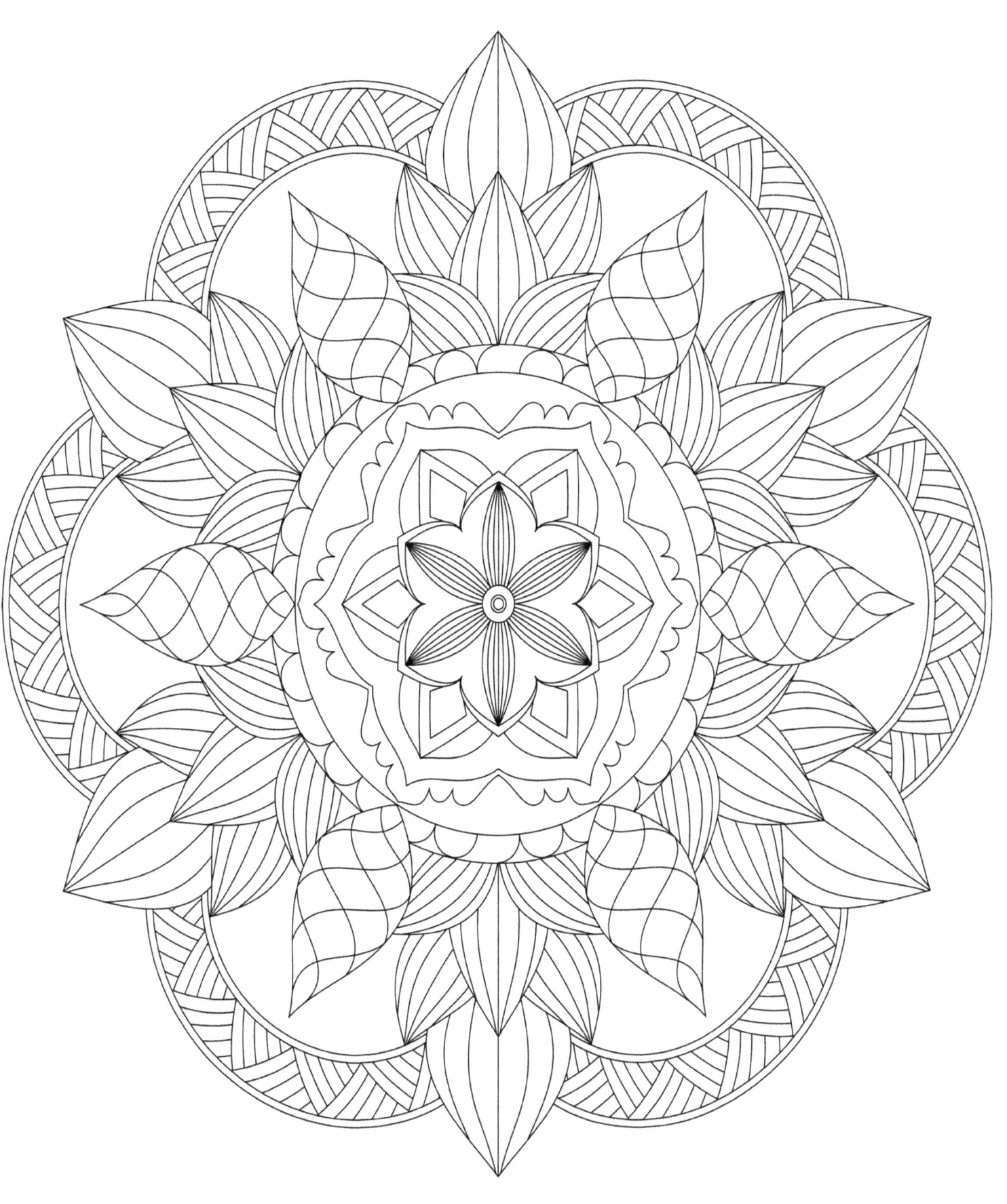

How Are You Feeling Today?

MENTAL HEALTH **PHYSICAL HEALTH**

positive	exhausted	healthy	ill
great	helpless	active	in pain
accomplished	hopeless	energetic	weight gain
frustrated	guilty	fatigued	weight loss
isolated	bothersome	hungry	thirsty
depressed	loveless	no appetite	nauseous
discouraged	ugly	insomnia	bloated
lonely	bored	achy	blockage

Notes: _____

_____

_____

_____

_____

_____

_____

_____

_____

_____

_____

_____

_____

_____

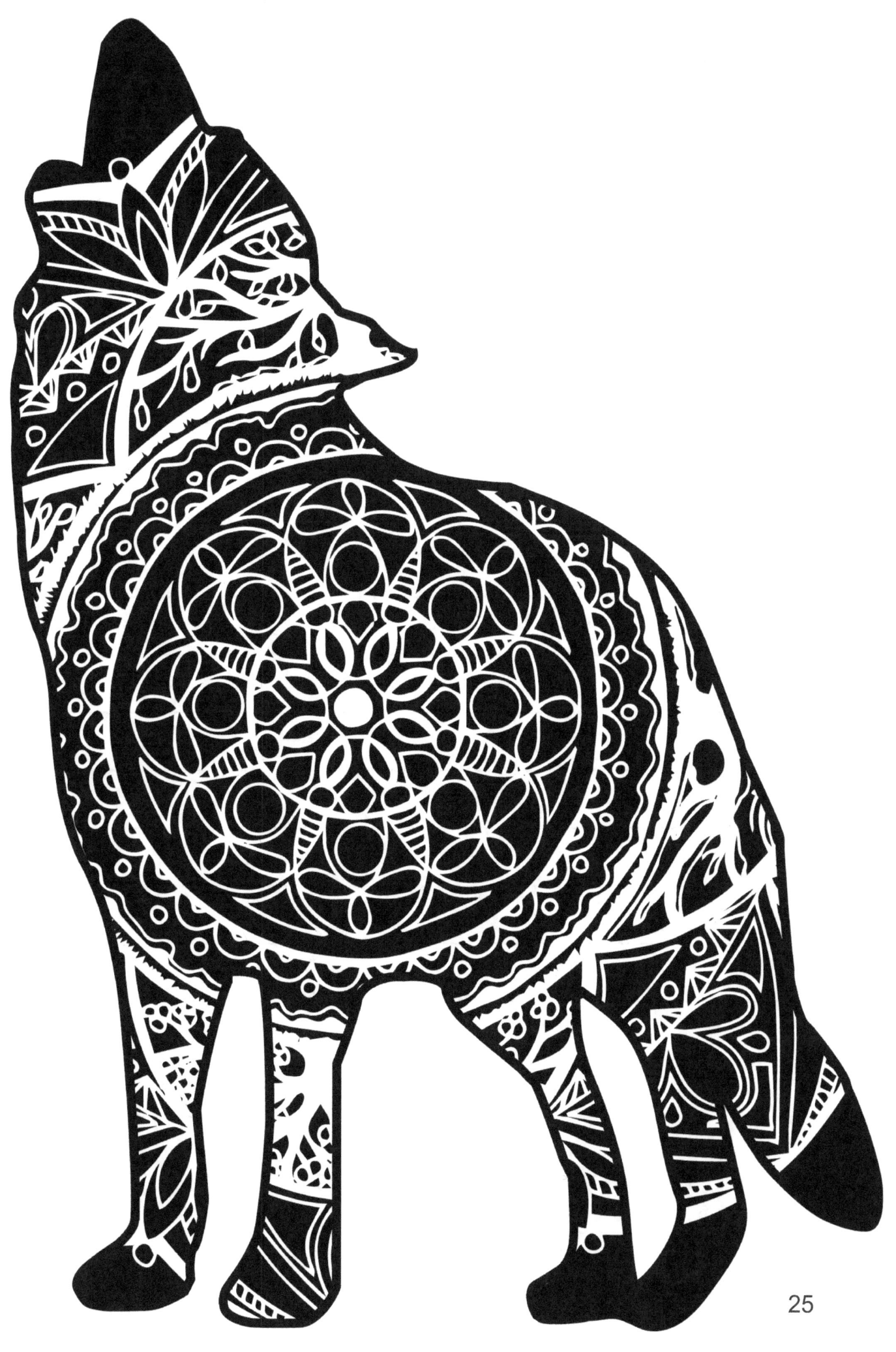

How Are You Feeling Today?

MENTAL HEALTH   **PHYSICAL HEALTH**

positive	exhausted	healthy	ill
great	helpless	active	in pain
accomplished	hopeless	energetic	weight gain
frustrated	guilty	fatigued	weight loss
isolated	bothersome	hungry	thirsty
depressed	loveless	no appetite	nauseous
discouraged	ugly	insomnia	bloated
lonely	bored	achy	blockage

Notes: _____

_____

_____

_____

_____

_____

_____

_____

_____

_____

_____

_____

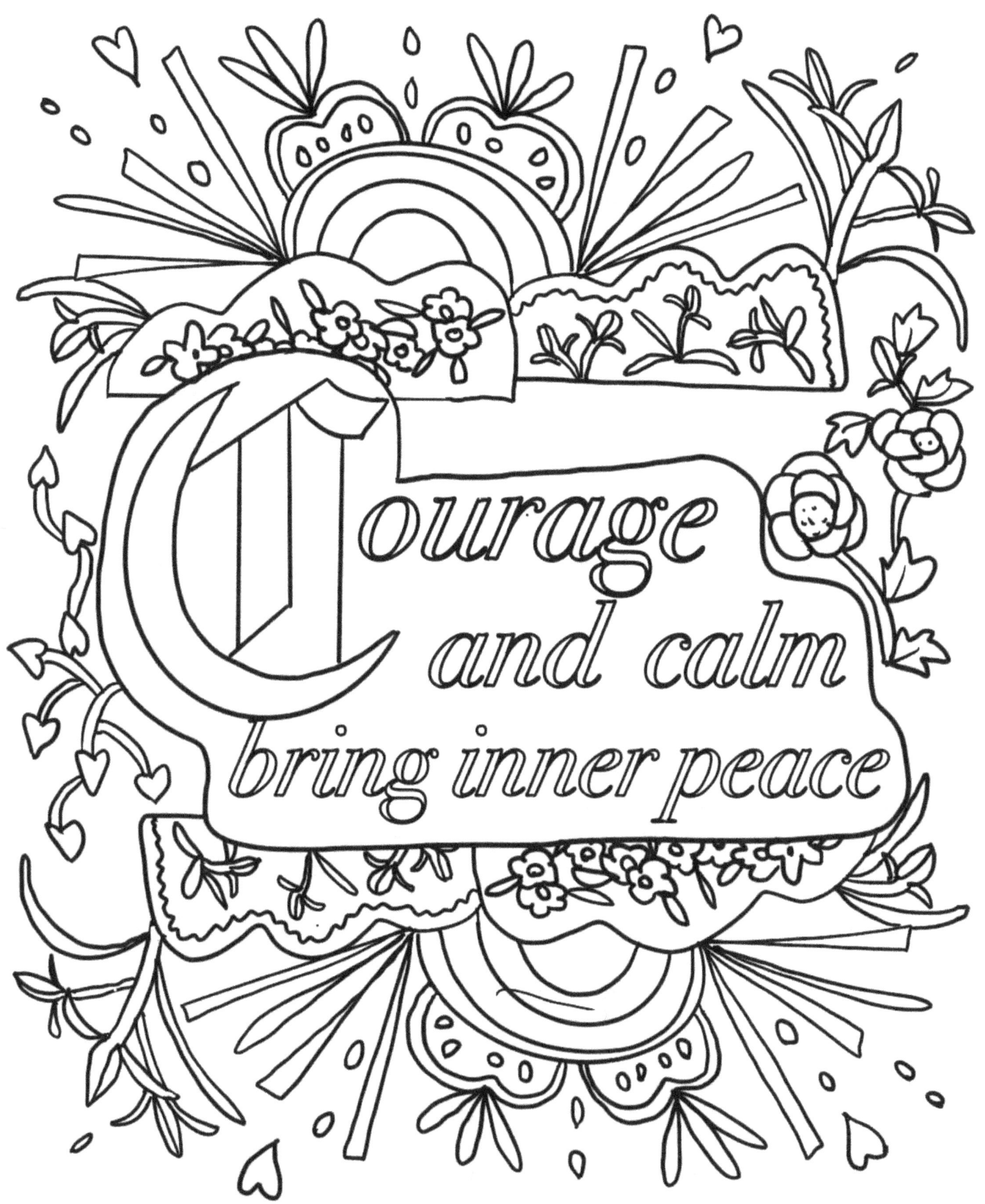

How Are You Feeling Today?

MENTAL HEALTH   **PHYSICAL HEALTH**

positive	exhausted	healthy	ill
great	helpless	active	in pain
accomplished	hopeless	energetic	weight gain
frustrated	guilty	fatigued	weight loss
isolated	bothersome	hungry	thirsty
depressed	loveless	no appetite	nauseous
discouraged	ugly	insomnia	bloated
lonely	bored	achy	blockage

Notes: _____

_____

_____

_____

_____

_____

_____

_____

_____

_____

_____

_____

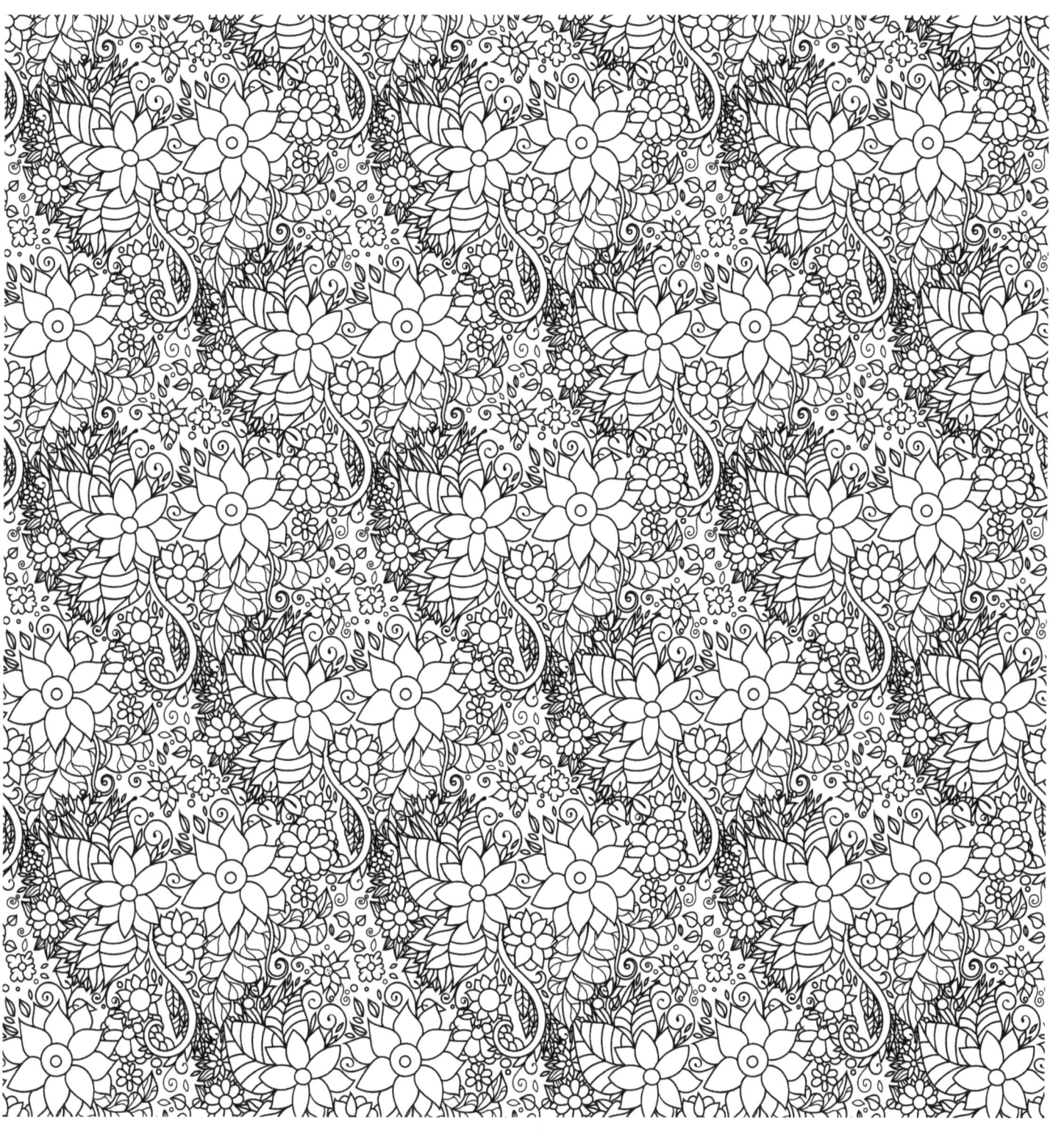

How Are You Feeling Today?

MENTAL HEALTH **PHYSICAL HEALTH**

positive	exhausted	healthy	ill
great	helpless	active	in pain
accomplished	hopeless	energetic	weight gain
frustrated	guilty	fatigued	weight loss
isolated	bothersome	hungry	thirsty
depressed	loveless	no appetite	nauseous
discouraged	ugly	insomnia	bloated
lonely	bored	achy	blockage

Notes: _____

_____

_____

_____

_____

_____

_____

_____

_____

_____

_____

_____

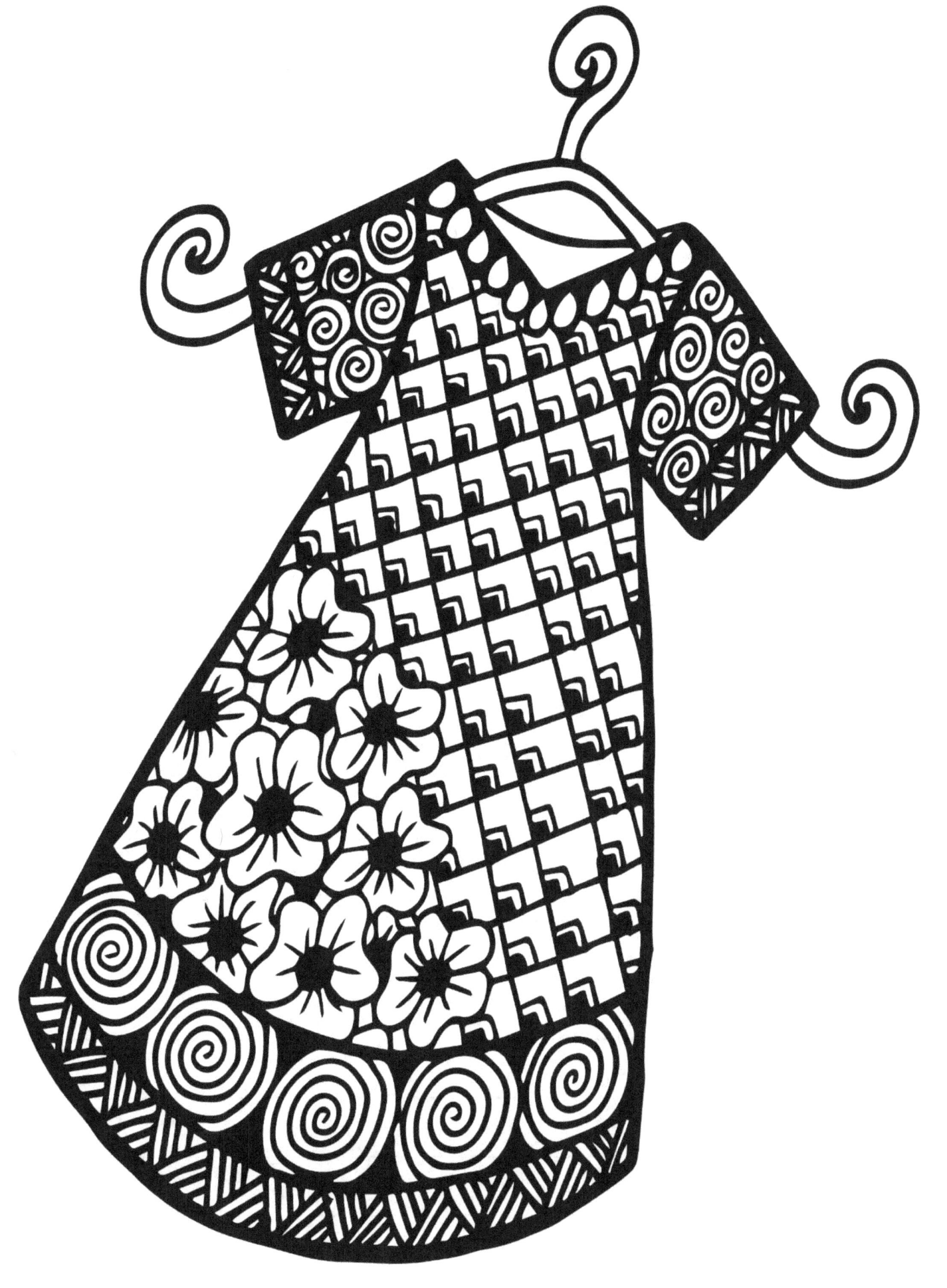

How Are You Feeling Today?

MENTAL HEALTH   **PHYSICAL HEALTH**

positive	exhausted	healthy	ill
great	helpless	active	in pain
accomplished	hopeless	energetic	weight gain
frustrated	guilty	fatigued	weight loss
isolated	bothersome	hungry	thirsty
depressed	loveless	no appetite	nauseous
discouraged	ugly	insomnia	bloated
lonely	bored	achy	blockage

Notes: _____

_____

_____

_____

_____

_____

_____

_____

_____

_____

_____

_____

_____

_____

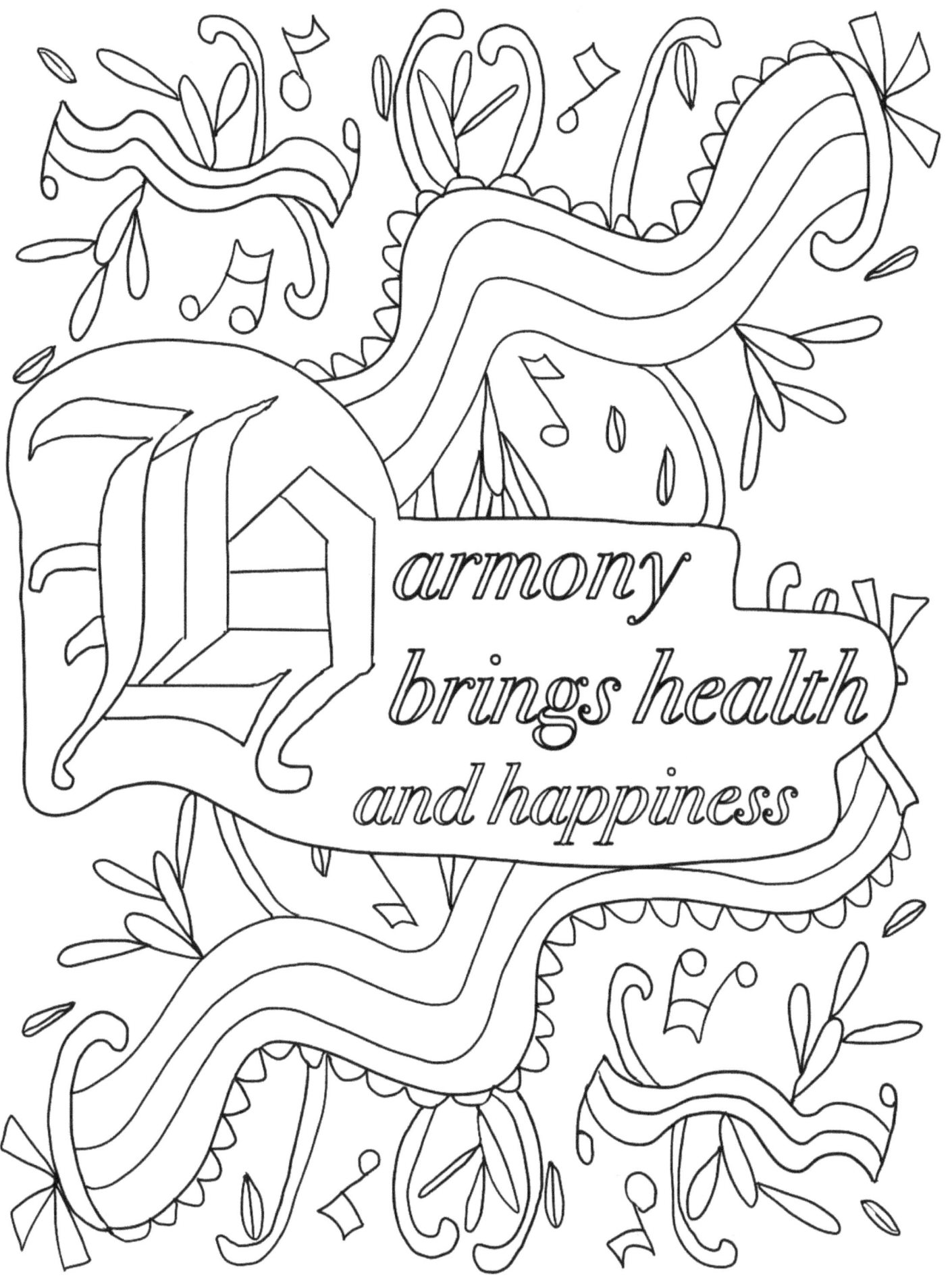

How Are You Feeling Today?

MENTAL HEALTH **PHYSICAL HEALTH**

positive	exhausted	healthy	ill
great	helpless	active	in pain
accomplished	hopeless	energetic	weight gain
frustrated	guilty	fatigued	weight loss
isolated	bothersome	hungry	thirsty
depressed	loveless	no appetite	nauseous
discouraged	ugly	insomnia	bloated
lonely	bored	achy	blockage

Notes: _____

_____

_____

_____

_____

_____

_____

_____

_____

_____

_____

_____

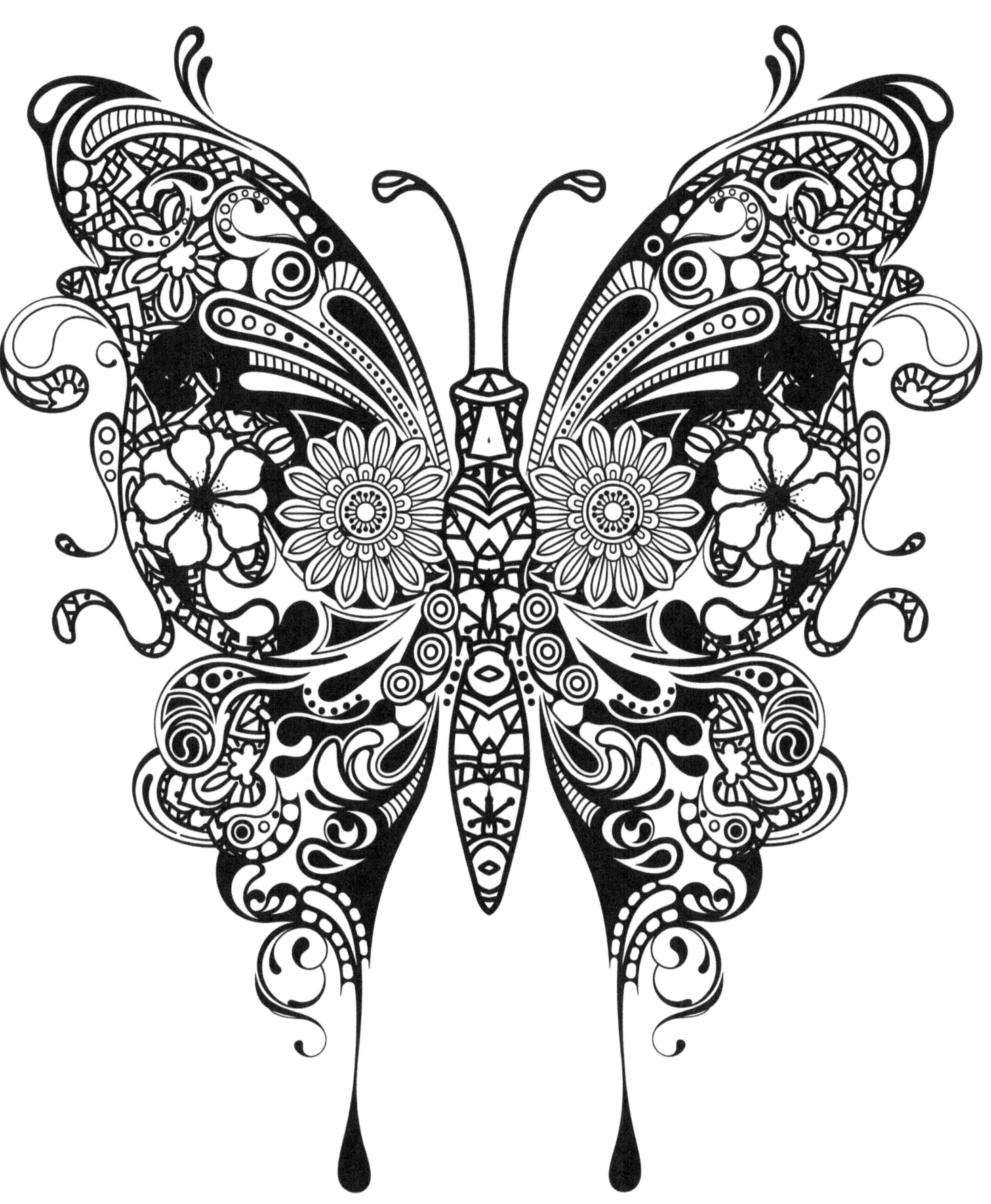

How Are You Feeling Today?

MENTAL HEALTH **PHYSICAL HEALTH**

positive	exhausted	healthy	ill
great	helpless	active	in pain
accomplished	hopeless	energetic	weight gain
frustrated	guilty	fatigued	weight loss
isolated	bothersome	hungry	thirsty
depressed	loveless	no appetite	nauseous
discouraged	ugly	insomnia	bloated
lonely	bored	achy	blockage

Notes: _____

_____

_____

_____

_____

_____

_____

_____

_____

_____

_____

_____

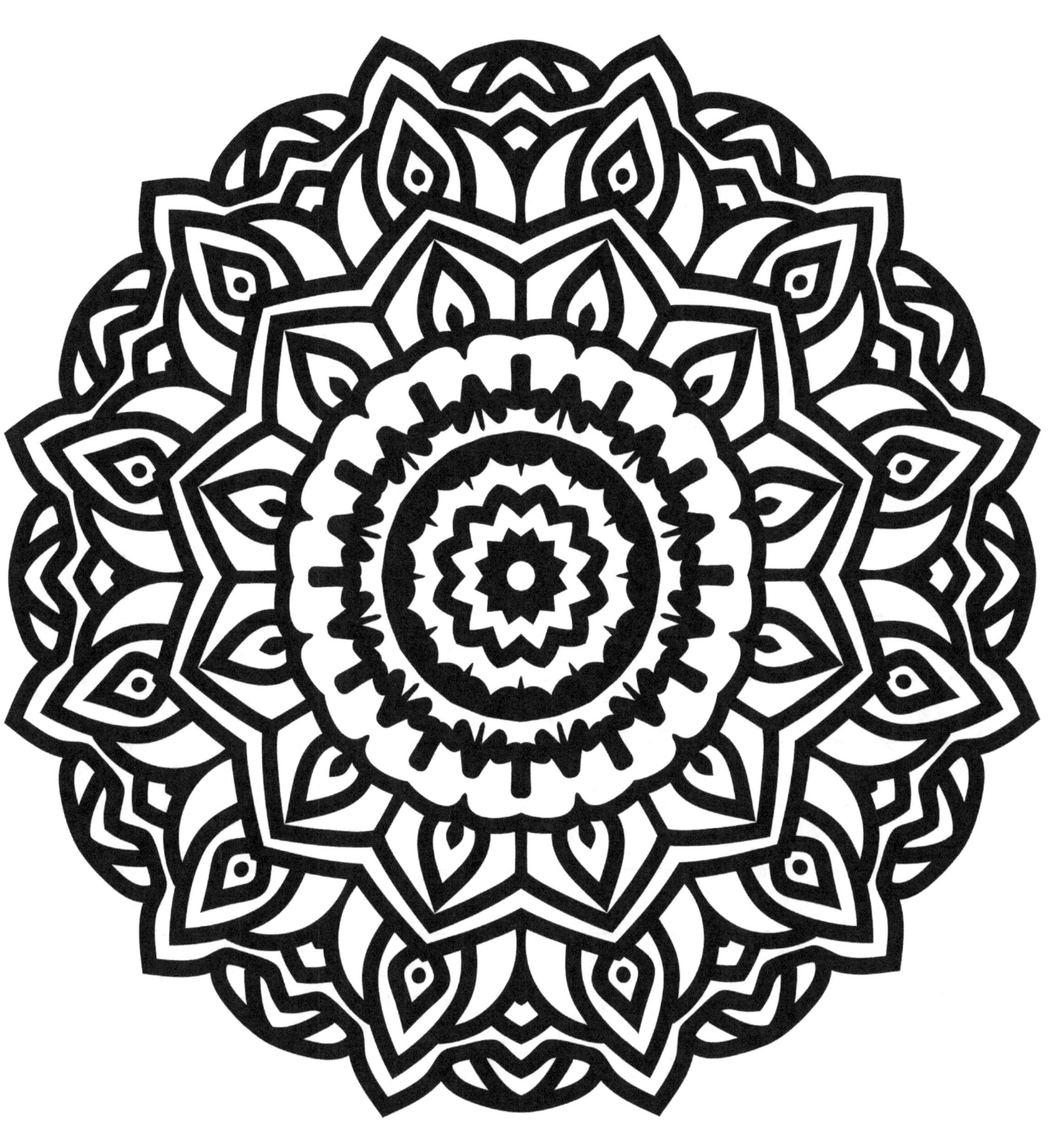

How Are You Feeling Today?

MENTAL HEALTH **PHYSICAL HEALTH**

positive	exhausted	healthy	ill
great	helpless	active	in pain
accomplished	hopeless	energetic	weight gain
frustrated	guilty	fatigued	weight loss
isolated	bothersome	hungry	thirsty
depressed	loveless	no appetite	nauseous
discouraged	ugly	insomnia	bloated
lonely	bored	achy	blockage

Notes: _____

_____

_____

_____

_____

_____

_____

_____

_____

_____

_____

_____

_____

_____

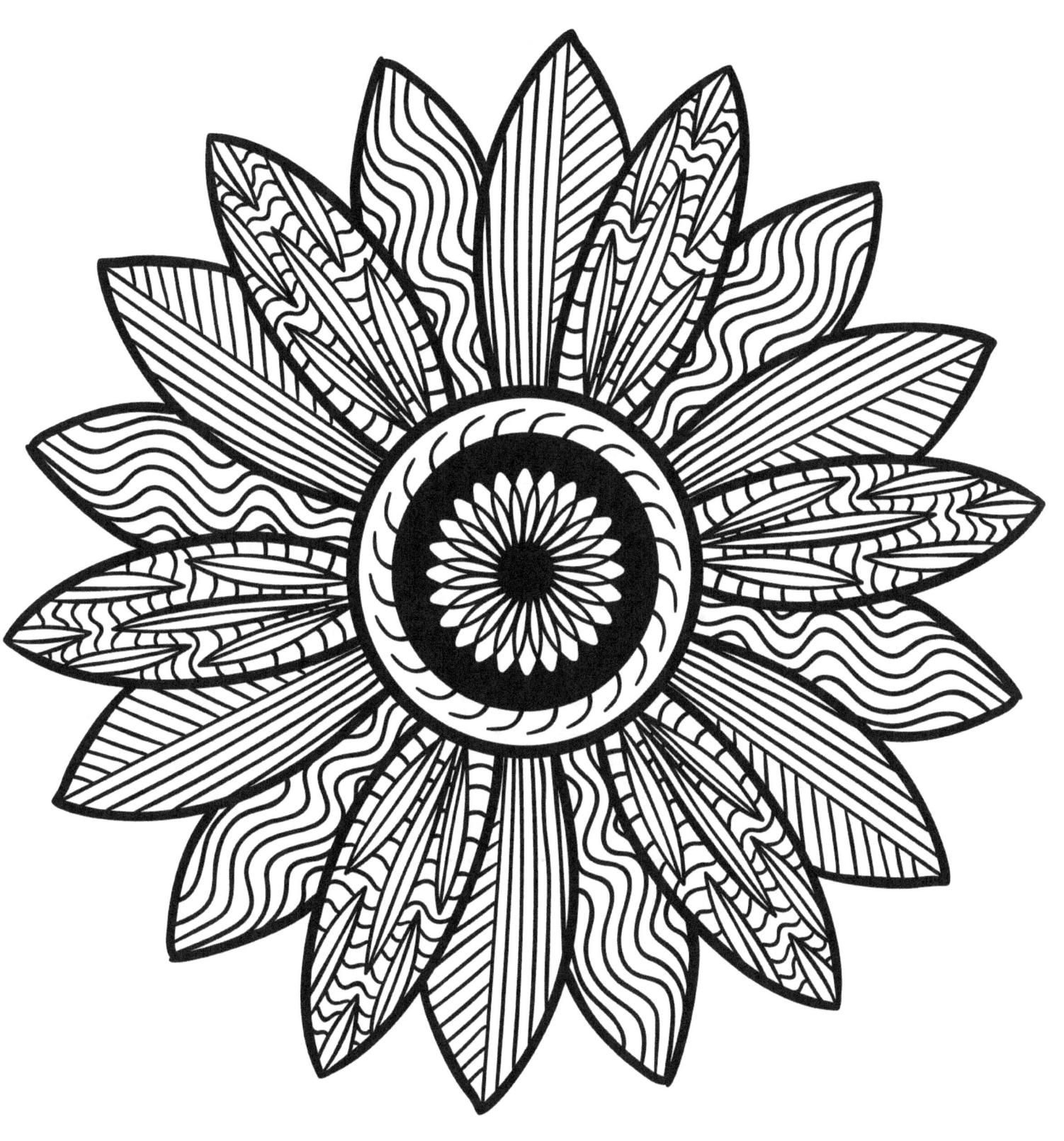

How Are You Feeling Today?

MENTAL HEALTH **PHYSICAL HEALTH**

positive	exhausted	healthy	ill
great	helpless	active	in pain
accomplished	hopeless	energetic	weight gain
frustrated	guilty	fatigued	weight loss
isolated	bothersome	hungry	thirsty
depressed	loveless	no appetite	nauseous
discouraged	ugly	insomnia	bloated
lonely	bored	achy	blockage

Notes: _____

_____

_____

_____

_____

_____

_____

_____

_____

_____

_____

_____

_____

_____

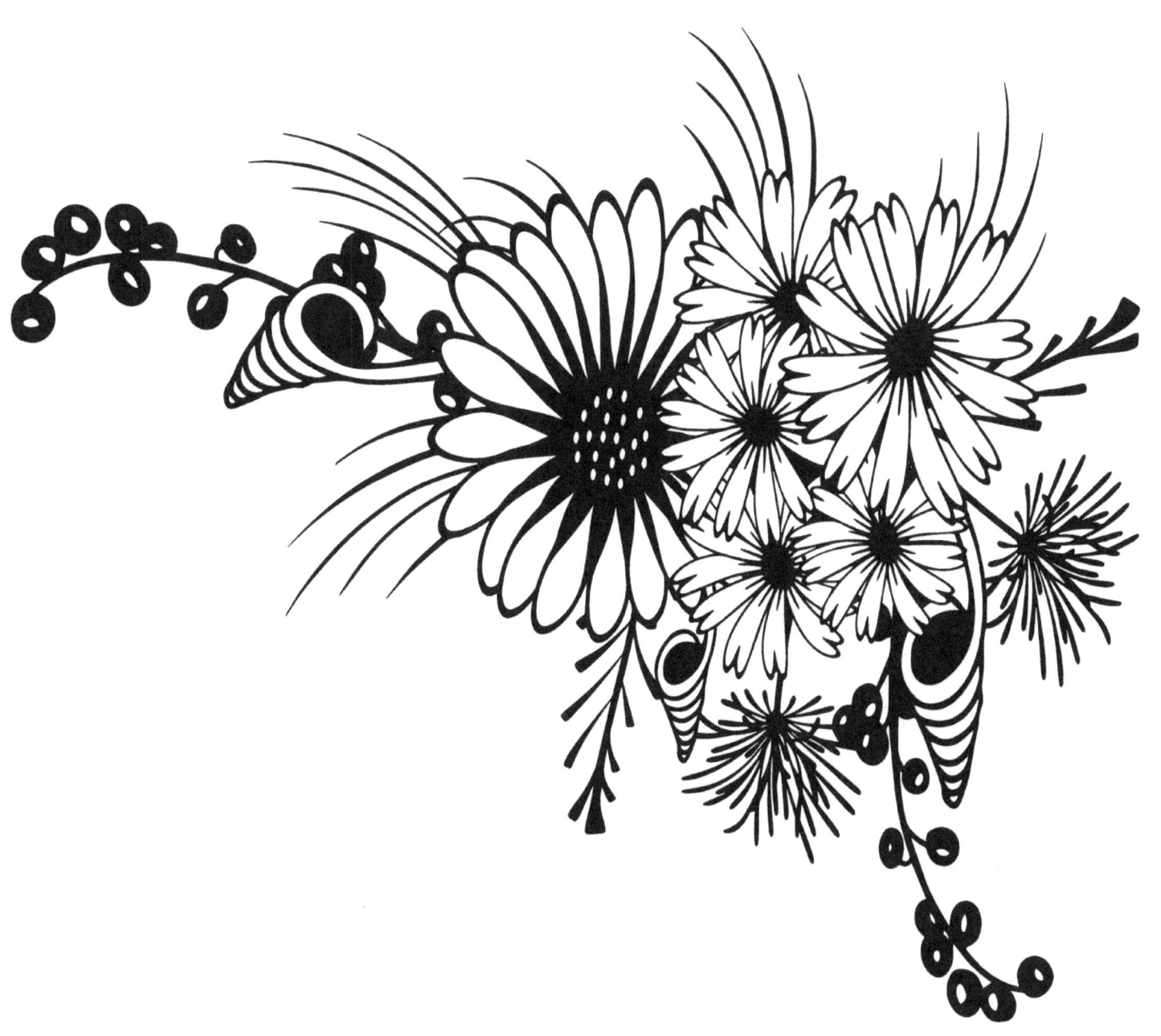

How Are You Feeling Today?

MENTAL HEALTH **PHYSICAL HEALTH**

positive	exhausted	healthy	ill
great	helpless	active	in pain
accomplished	hopeless	energetic	weight gain
frustrated	guilty	fatigued	weight loss
isolated	bothersome	hungry	thirsty
depressed	loveless	no appetite	nauseous
discouraged	ugly	insomnia	bloated
lonely	bored	achy	blockage

Notes: _____

_____

_____

_____

_____

_____

_____

_____

_____

_____

_____

_____

_____

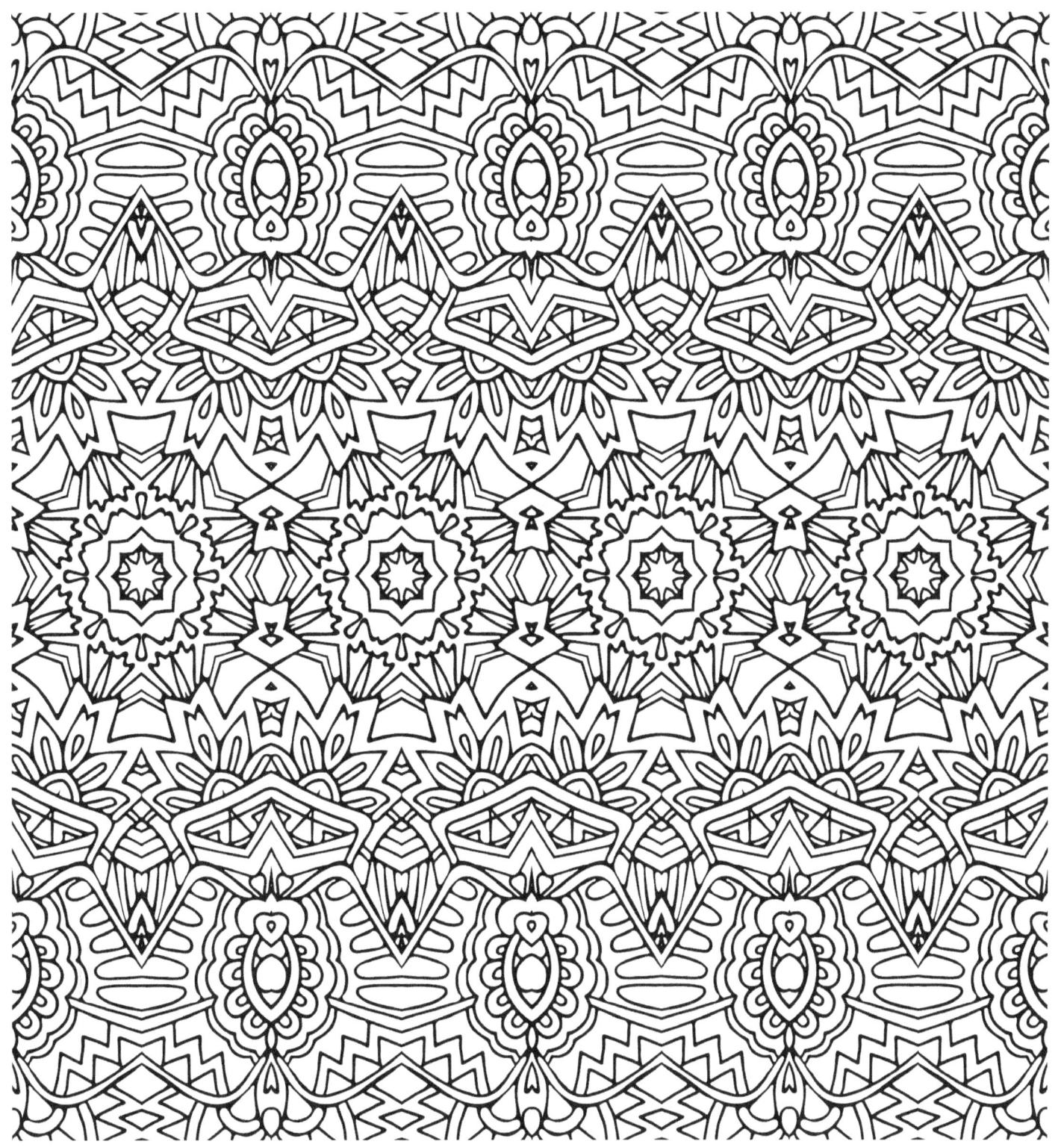

How Are You Feeling Today?

MENTAL HEALTH **PHYSICAL HEALTH**

positive	exhausted	healthy	ill
great	helpless	active	in pain
accomplished	hopeless	energetic	weight gain
frustrated	guilty	fatigued	weight loss
isolated	bothersome	hungry	thirsty
depressed	loveless	no appetite	nauseous
discouraged	ugly	insomnia	bloated
lonely	bored	achy	blockage

Notes: _____

_____

_____

_____

_____

_____

_____

_____

_____

_____

_____

_____

_____

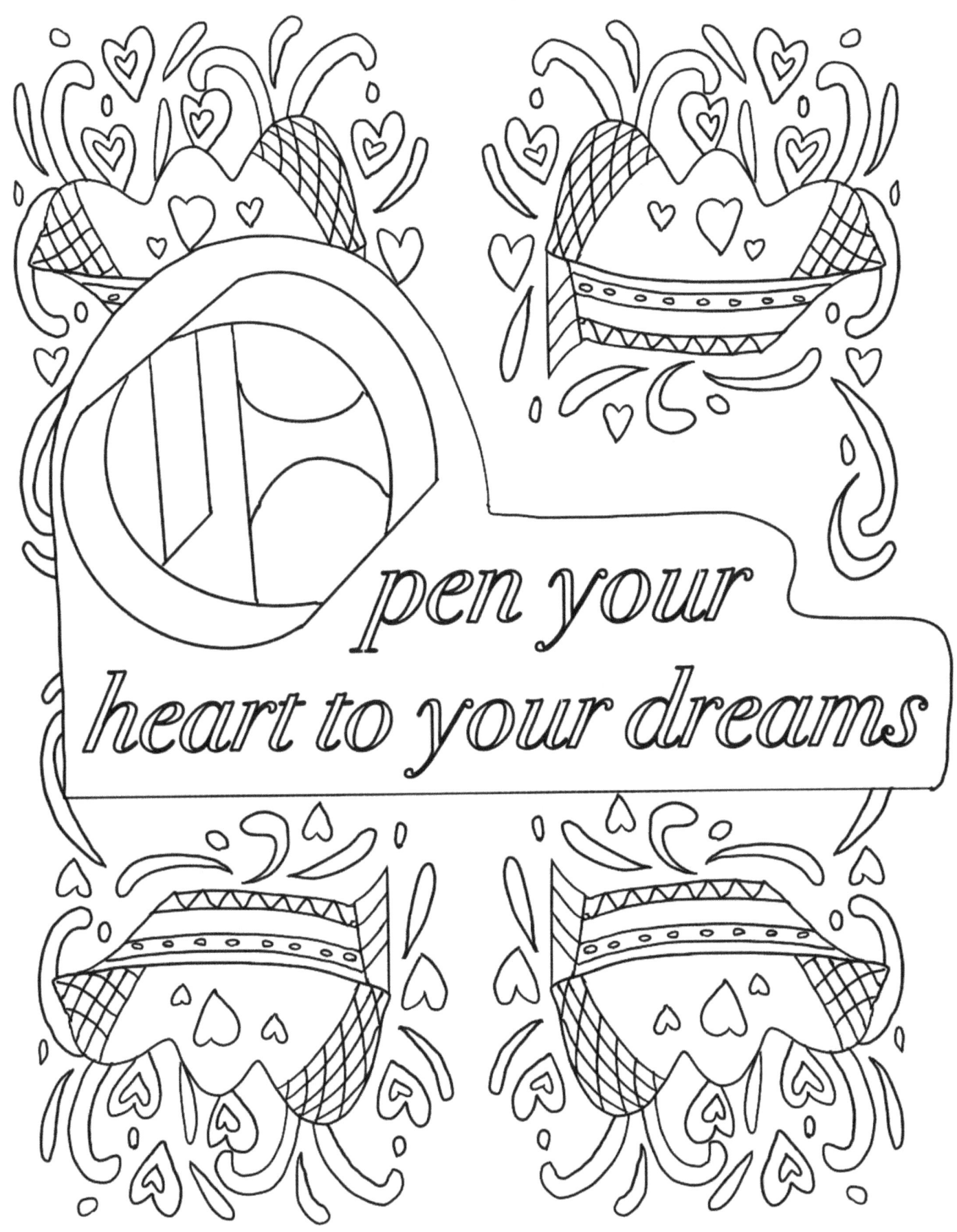

How Are You Feeling Today?

MENTAL HEALTH **PHYSICAL HEALTH**

	positive		exhausted		healthy		ill
	great		helpless		active		in pain
	accomplished		hopeless		energetic		weight gain
	frustrated		guilty		fatigued		weight loss
	isolated		bothersome		hungry		thirsty
	depressed		loveless		no appetite		nauseous
	discouraged		ugly		insomnia		bloated
	lonely		bored		achy		blockage

Notes: _____

_____

_____

_____

_____

_____

_____

_____

_____

_____

_____

_____

_____

_____

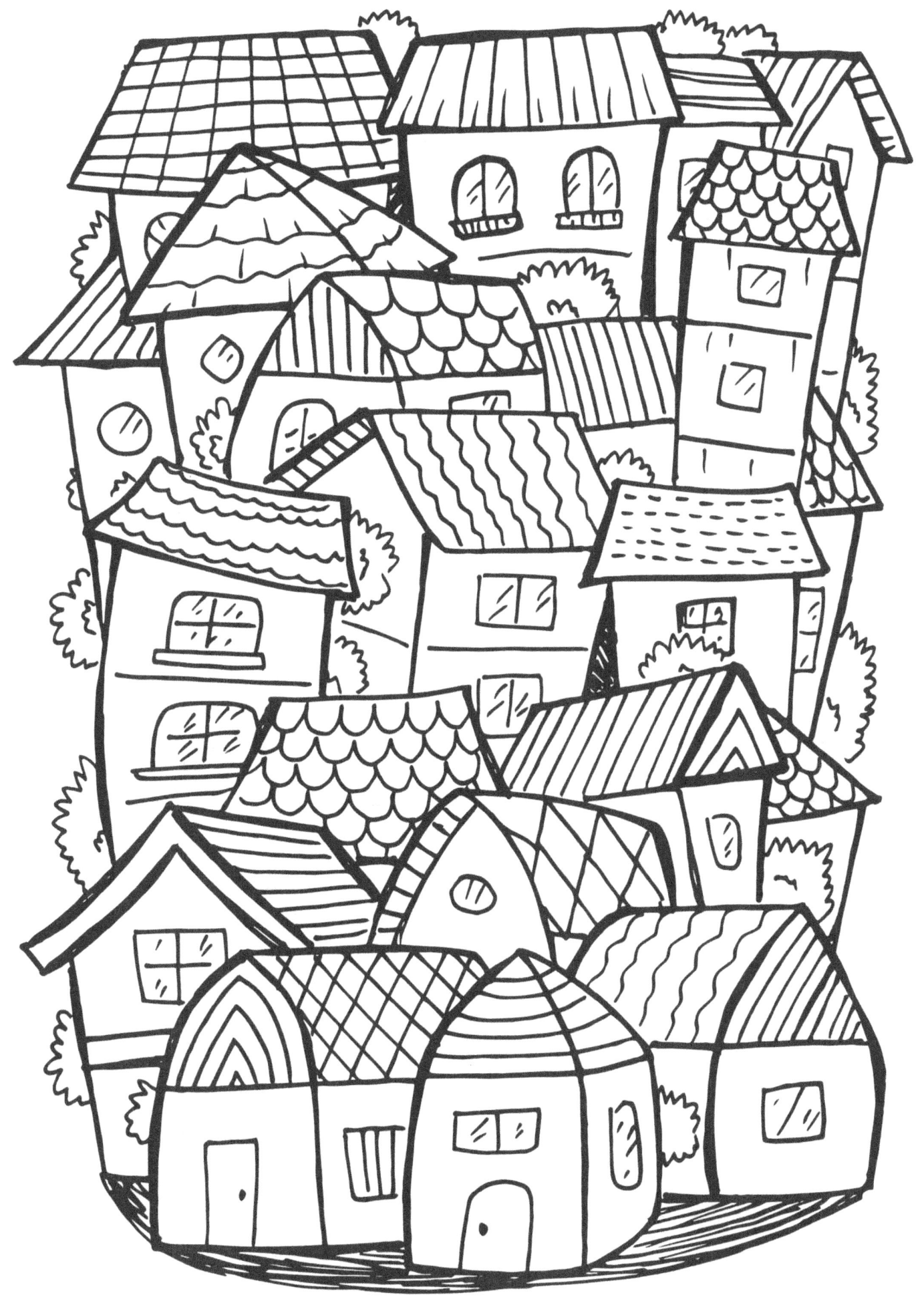

How Are You Feeling Today?

MENTAL HEALTH   **PHYSICAL HEALTH**

positive	exhausted	healthy	ill
great	helpless	active	in pain
accomplished	hopeless	energetic	weight gain
frustrated	guilty	fatigued	weight loss
isolated	bothersome	hungry	thirsty
depressed	loveless	no appetite	nauseous
discouraged	ugly	insomnia	bloated
lonely	bored	achy	blockage

Notes: _____

_____

_____

_____

_____

_____

_____

_____

_____

_____

_____

_____

_____

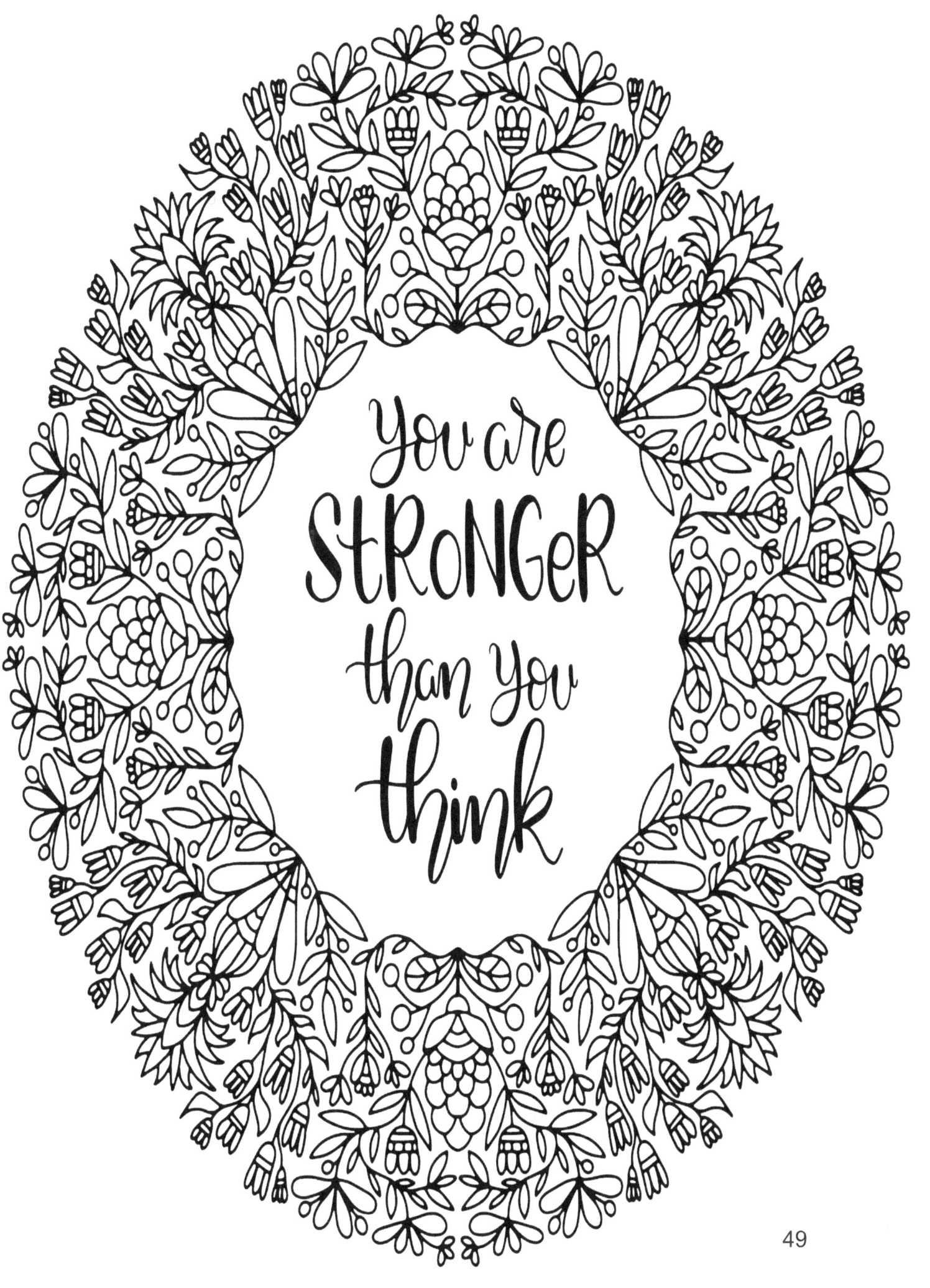

How Are You Feeling Today?

MENTAL HEALTH **PHYSICAL HEALTH**

positive	exhausted	healthy	ill
great	helpless	active	in pain
accomplished	hopeless	energetic	weight gain
frustrated	guilty	fatigued	weight loss
isolated	bothersome	hungry	thirsty
depressed	loveless	no appetite	nauseous
discouraged	ugly	insomnia	bloated
lonely	bored	achy	blockage

Notes: _____

_____

_____

_____

_____

_____

_____

_____

_____

_____

_____

_____

_____

_____

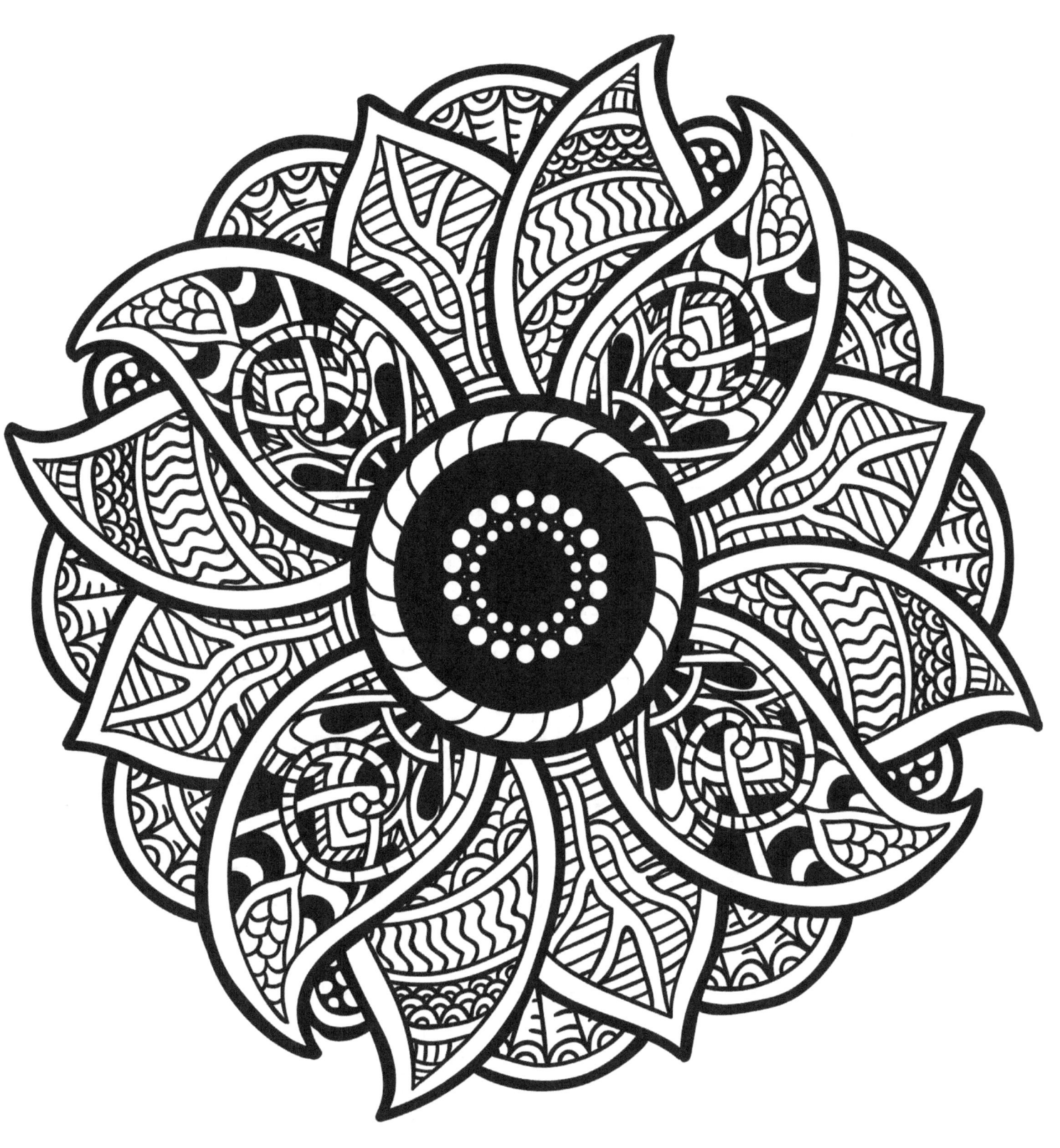

How Are You Feeling Today?

MENTAL HEALTH **PHYSICAL HEALTH**

positive	exhausted	healthy	ill
great	helpless	active	in pain
accomplished	hopeless	energetic	weight gain
frustrated	guilty	fatigued	weight loss
isolated	bothersome	hungry	thirsty
depressed	loveless	no appetite	nauseous
discouraged	ugly	insomnia	bloated
lonely	bored	achy	blockage

Notes: _____

_____
_____
_____
_____
_____
_____
_____
_____
_____
_____
_____
_____
_____
_____

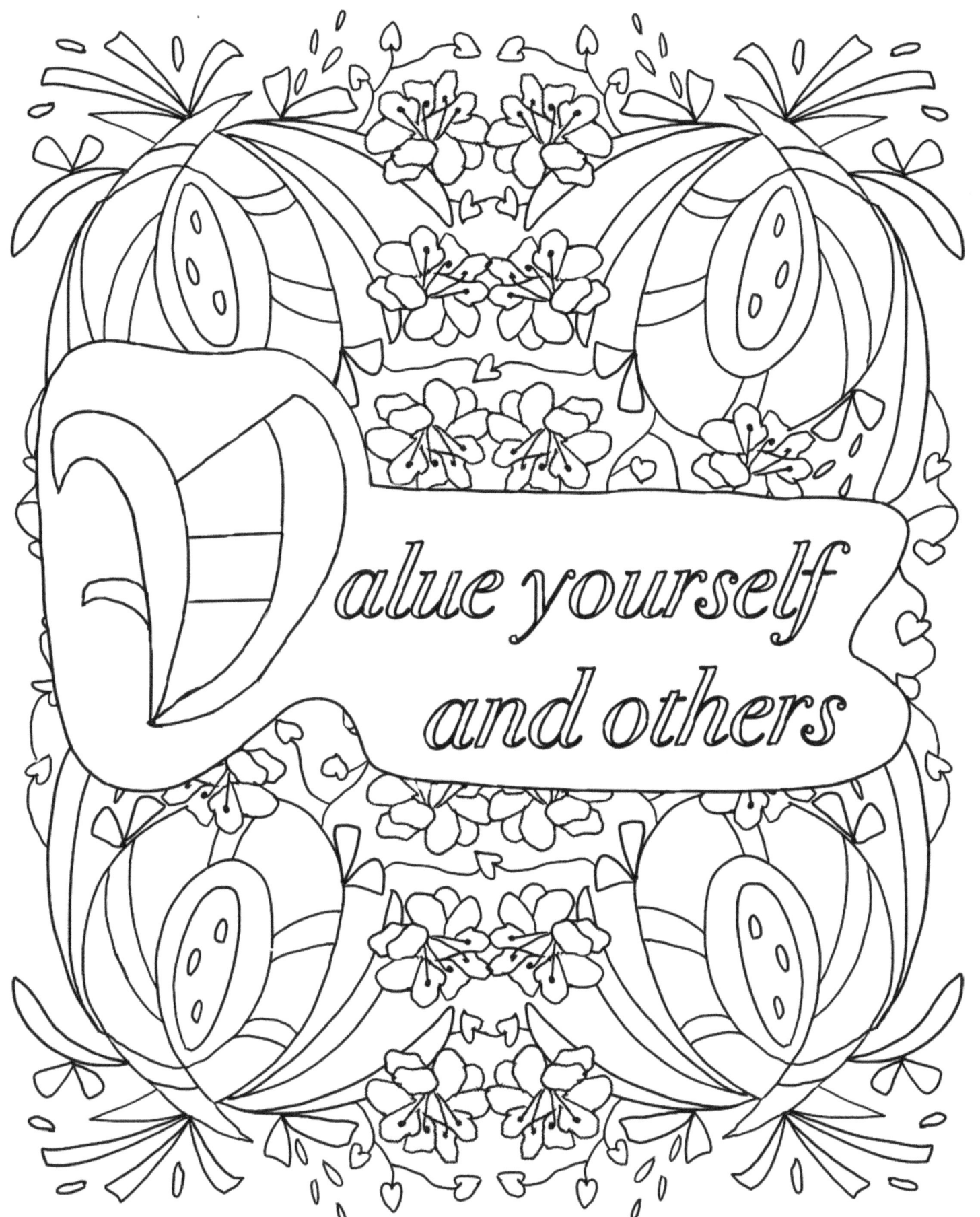

How Are You Feeling Today?

MENTAL HEALTH   **PHYSICAL HEALTH**

positive	exhausted	healthy	ill
great	helpless	active	in pain
accomplished	hopeless	energetic	weight gain
frustrated	guilty	fatigued	weight loss
isolated	bothersome	hungry	thirsty
depressed	loveless	no appetite	nauseous
discouraged	ugly	insomnia	bloated
lonely	bored	achy	blockage

Notes: _____

_____

_____

_____

_____

_____

_____

_____

_____

_____

_____

_____

_____

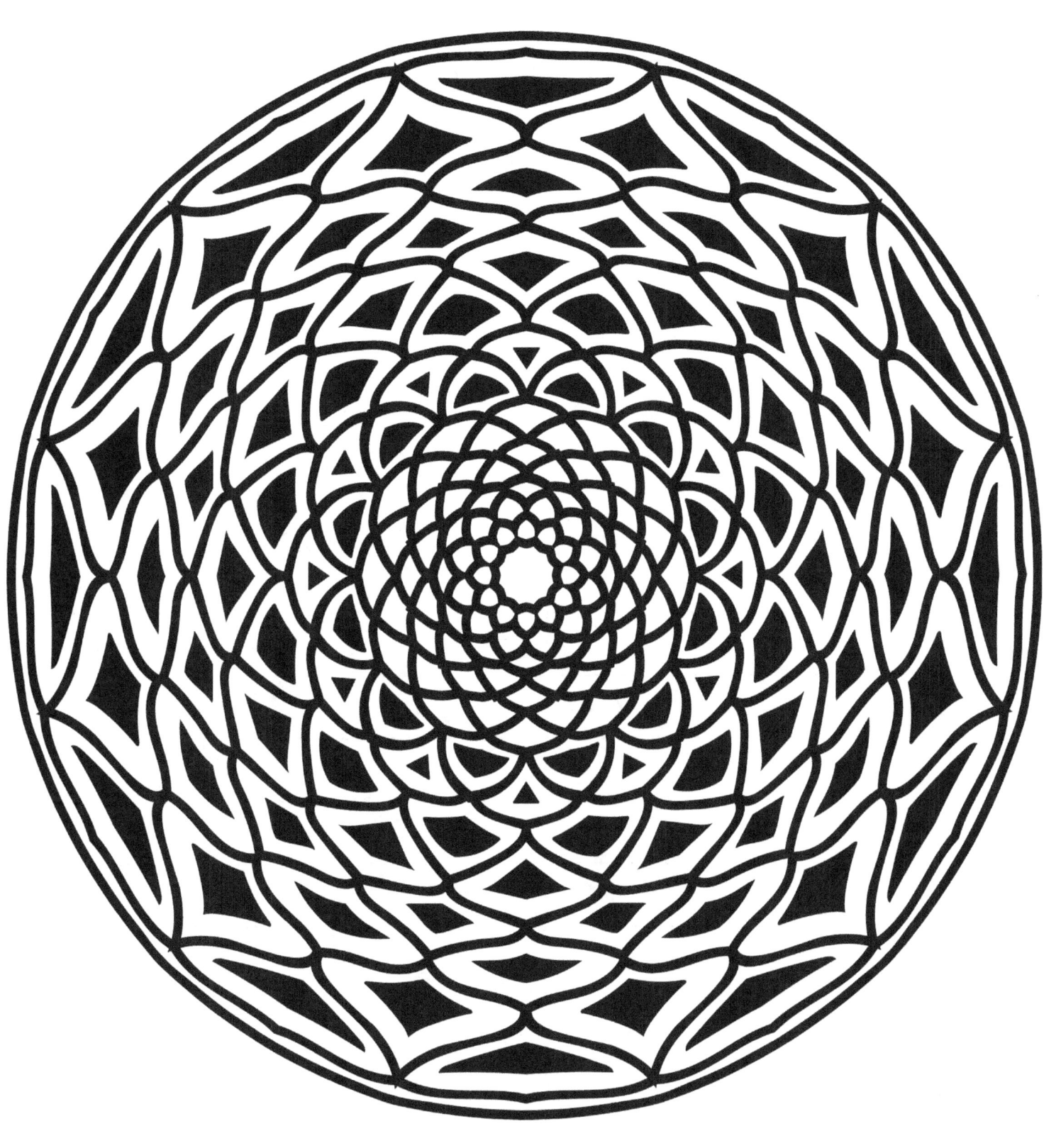

How Are You Feeling Today?

MENTAL HEALTH **PHYSICAL HEALTH**

positive	exhausted	healthy	ill
great	helpless	active	in pain
accomplished	hopeless	energetic	weight gain
frustrated	guilty	fatigued	weight loss
isolated	bothersome	hungry	thirsty
depressed	loveless	no appetite	nauseous
discouraged	ugly	insomnia	bloated
lonely	bored	achy	blockage

Notes: _____

_____

_____

_____

_____

_____

_____

_____

_____

_____

_____

_____

_____

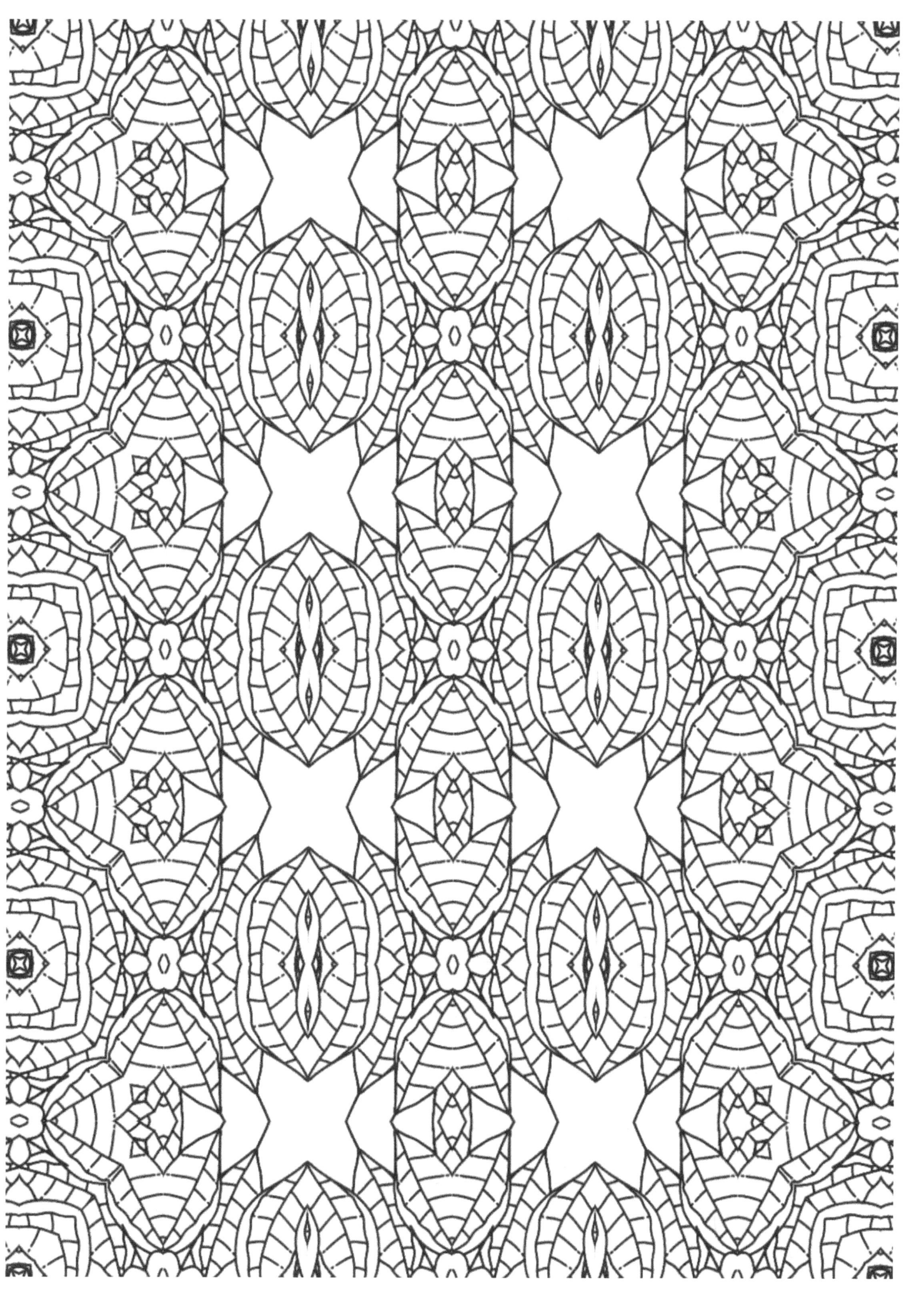

How Are You Feeling Today?

MENTAL HEALTH **PHYSICAL HEALTH**

positive	exhausted	healthy	ill
great	helpless	active	in pain
accomplished	hopeless	energetic	weight gain
frustrated	guilty	fatigued	weight loss
isolated	bothersome	hungry	thirsty
depressed	loveless	no appetite	nauseous
discouraged	ugly	insomnia	bloated
lonely	bored	achy	blockage

Notes: _____

_____

_____

_____

_____

_____

_____

_____

_____

_____

_____

_____

_____

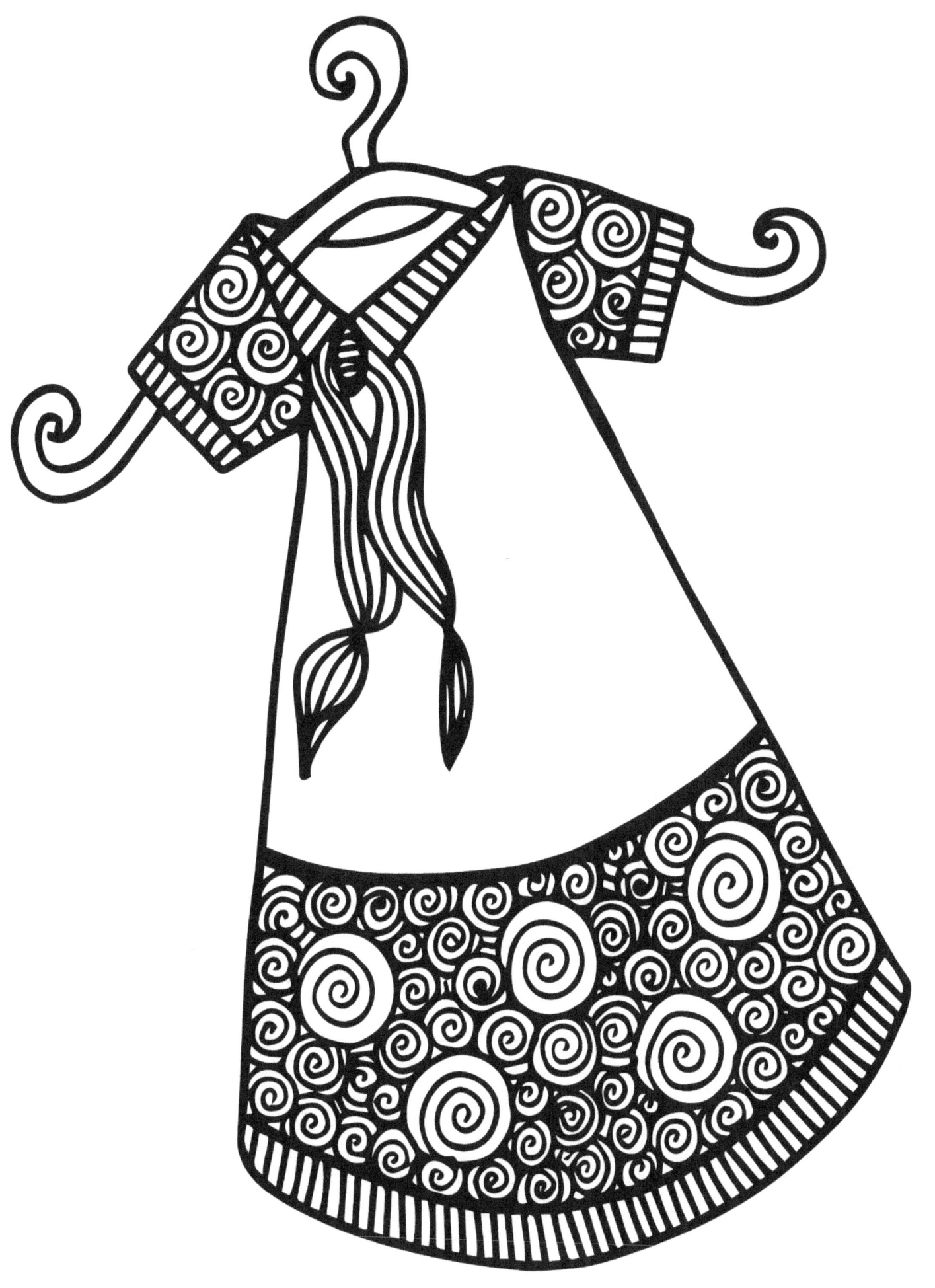

How Are You Feeling Today?

MENTAL HEALTH **PHYSICAL HEALTH**

positive	exhausted	healthy	ill
great	helpless	active	in pain
accomplished	hopeless	energetic	weight gain
frustrated	guilty	fatigued	weight loss
isolated	bothersome	hungry	thirsty
depressed	loveless	no appetite	nauseous
discouraged	ugly	insomnia	bloated
lonely	bored	achy	blockage

Notes: _____

_____

_____

_____

_____

_____

_____

_____

_____

_____

_____

_____

_____

_____

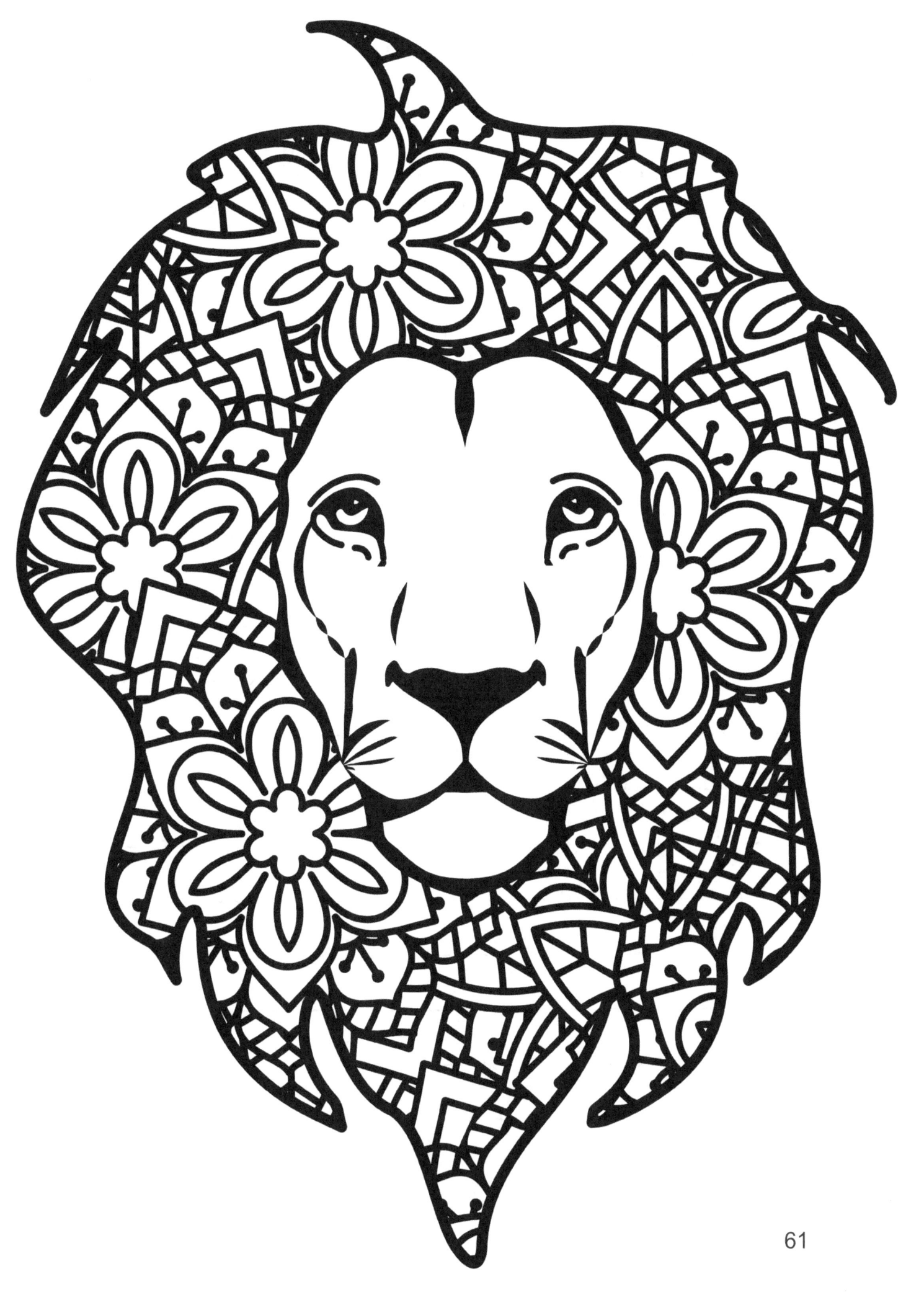

How Are You Feeling Today?

MENTAL HEALTH **PHYSICAL HEALTH**

	positive		exhausted		healthy		ill
	great		helpless		active		in pain
	accomplished		hopeless		energetic		weight gain
	frustrated		guilty		fatigued		weight loss
	isolated		bothersome		hungry		thirsty
	depressed		loveless		no appetite		nauseous
	discouraged		ugly		insomnia		bloated
	lonely		bored		achy		blockage

Notes: _____

_____

_____

_____

_____

_____

_____

_____

_____

_____

_____

_____

_____

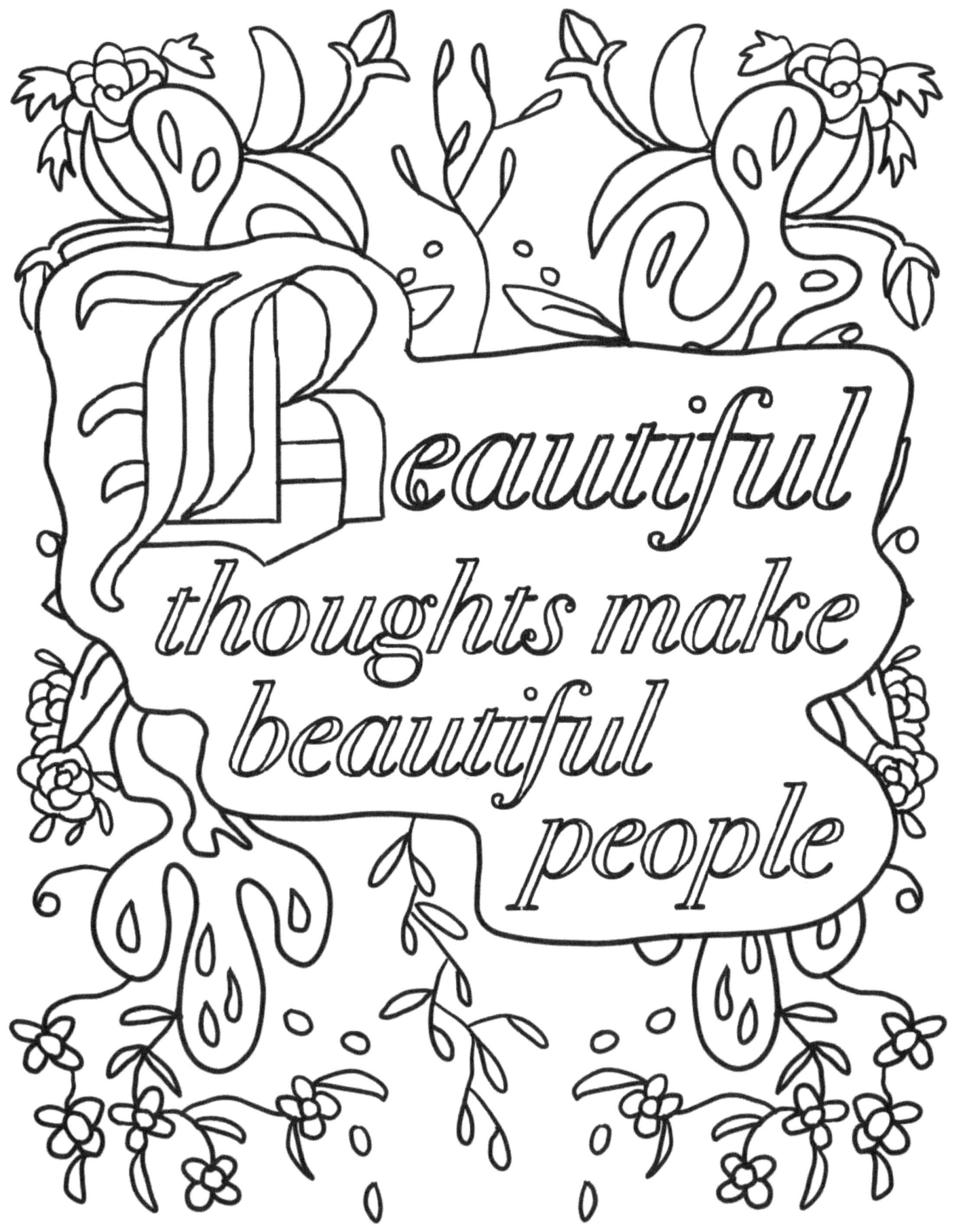

How Are You Feeling Today?

MENTAL HEALTH **PHYSICAL HEALTH**

positive	exhausted	healthy	ill
great	helpless	active	in pain
accomplished	hopeless	energetic	weight gain
frustrated	guilty	fatigued	weight loss
isolated	bothersome	hungry	thirsty
depressed	loveless	no appetite	nauseous
discouraged	ugly	insomnia	bloated
lonely	bored	achy	blockage

Notes: _____

_____

_____

_____

_____

_____

_____

_____

_____

_____

_____

_____

_____

COLON CANCER

ANSWERS ON PAGE 75

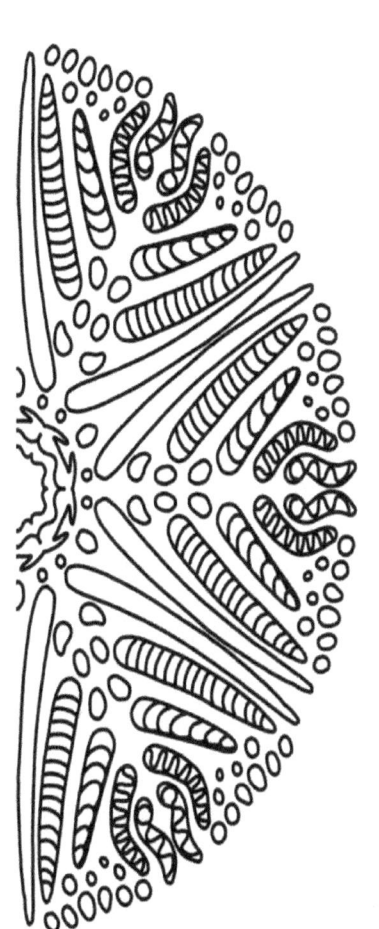

```
A I C A R E G I V E R E D X G R S N D L
N Q S Y E L O S T O M Y S U R V I V O R
E X U Z U Y A H U Y M O T S O E L I G Z
P T N E M E G A N A M N I A P S S R W C
G Z H G A B A M O T S O O J E F E O E O
W E M I S T R W V H Y D M R J C W M G L
O R R X B T W E O I V P E E N B R O E O
U A H M B D O L C J Y A H A G J U S Y R
N C C N H I L M D N Y I C A S A A E T E
D F X Z O I S I A G A N M S Q E K Y R C
N L E Y S I N W O R O C E O S D M A O T
U E X T T P T L E L E N L I O O F S E A
R S E D C I O A O P E V D E T R I L A L
S R R U A C S C X R Y S E S W T H A I I
E B C C N V U E A A N T O R I O P T W L
P N I O H W S W B H L L D L S J B I A C
E I S W O O A W O O O E O O S A M P D B
E R E S P W Z R Q C I C R H O G L S M P
L W D I E T C M U T C E R F I L L O P M
S I N S P I R A T I O N Z E A D B H N K
```

WORD LIST:

- COLON CANCER
- PAIN
- COLORECTAL
- PAIN MANAGEMENT
- HOSPITAL
- ONCOLOGY
- WOUND NURSE
- IBD
- SLEEP
- AWARENESS
- STOMA BAG
- OSTOMY SURVIVOR
- OBESITY
- INSPIRATION
- HOPE
- CHEMO
- CAREGIVER
- ILEOSTOMY
- COLOSTOMY
- RECTUM
- BOWEL CANCER
- CROHNS DISEASE
- COLITIS
- BATHROOM
- STOMA REVERSAL
- BLOOD TYPE
- LEAKAGE
- HOLLISTER
- RELAXATION
- SELF CARE
- DIET
- EXERCISE

© We Survived Publishing

How Are You Feeling Today?

MENTAL HEALTH   **PHYSICAL HEALTH**

positive	exhausted	healthy	ill
great	helpless	active	in pain
accomplished	hopeless	energetic	weight gain
frustrated	guilty	fatigued	weight loss
isolated	bothersome	hungry	thirsty
depressed	loveless	no appetite	nauseous
discouraged	ugly	insomnia	bloated
lonely	bored	achy	blockage

Notes: _____

_____

_____

_____

_____

_____

_____

_____

_____

_____

_____

_____

_____

_____

CANCER SCRAMBLE #1

ANSWERS ON PAGE 77

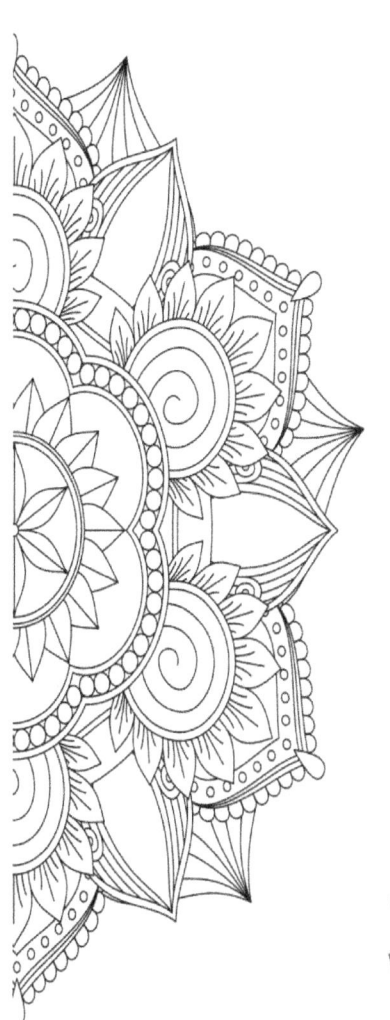

```
C Y A M O N I C R A C F B O S
N G P F M A R G O M M A M L Y
O T B A R E T E M A I D L I M
I T C A R T E V I T S E G I D
T N B Y S E D D R C C I H S C
A A F A N W H E O D N T Y Y A
I C C R G S M T O O W F B M T
D S M X I I T O O L I R P S
A I Y X S X L A R M O B Q T C
R R Y S R B U G G P E A L O A
P M I Q E C Q E S E B H B M N
H O W T C U X Y M D S S C S W
N M I X N P P R O G N O S I S
Q H B Q A Y M A L I G N A N T
W T L M C H O H A D R O M U T
```

WORD LIST:

BLOOD	MRI SCAN	TUMOR	DIGESTIVE TRACT
CARCINOMA	PROGNOSIS	WHITEBLOOD CELLS	GROWTH
CAT SCAN	XRAY	REMISSION	BIOPSY
MALIGNANT	CHEMOTHERAPY	DIAMETER	CANCER SIGNS
MAMMOGRAM	RADIATION	STAGES	SYMPTOMS

© We Survived Publishing

How Are You Feeling Today?

MENTAL HEALTH **PHYSICAL HEALTH**

positive	exhausted	healthy	ill
great	helpless	active	in pain
accomplished	hopeless	energetic	weight gain
frustrated	guilty	fatigued	weight loss
isolated	bothersome	hungry	thirsty
depressed	loveless	no appetite	nauseous
discouraged	ugly	insomnia	bloated
lonely	bored	achy	blockage

Notes: _____

_____

_____

_____

_____

_____

_____

_____

_____

_____

_____

_____

_____

THE BODY

ANSWERS ON PAGE 79

```
            K D C                 E S I
          N L R N E             S E N K C
        H I S Y U E S       L S T U S F H
        E K G G M E E I T E L E X S T
        A S N E Y P S L S S V I E G E
        R O U E A N H T P R A I A A E
        T J L U O R I N E S R E T N T
        W J T X N S N O A R V R K
        B S L E S S E V D O O L B
          L S S N R O Y W E X T
            A E H C A M O T S
              D N T R A E H
                D O C F E
                  E B R
                    R
```

WORD LIST:

SKIN	LYMPH NODES	TONSILS	EYES
NAILS	STOMACH	LUNGS	EARS
BONES	INTESTINES	HEART	HEART
NERVES	SPLEEN	BLADDER	TONGUE
BLOOD VESSELS	OVARIES	BREAST	TEETH

© We Survived Publishing

How Are You Feeling Today?

MENTAL HEALTH **PHYSICAL HEALTH**

☐	positive	☐	exhausted	☐	healthy	☐	ill
☐	great	☐	helpless	☐	active	☐	in pain
☐	accomplished	☐	hopeless	☐	energetic	☐	weight gain
☐	frustrated	☐	guilty	☐	fatigued	☐	weight loss
☐	isolated	☐	bothersome	☐	hungry	☐	thirsty
☐	depressed	☐	loveless	☐	no appetite	☐	nauseous
☐	discouraged	☐	ugly	☐	insomnia	☐	bloated
☐	lonely	☐	bored	☐	achy	☐	blockage

Notes: _____

_____

_____

_____

_____

_____

_____

_____

_____

_____

_____

_____

CANCER SCRAMBLE #2

ANSWERS ON PAGE 81

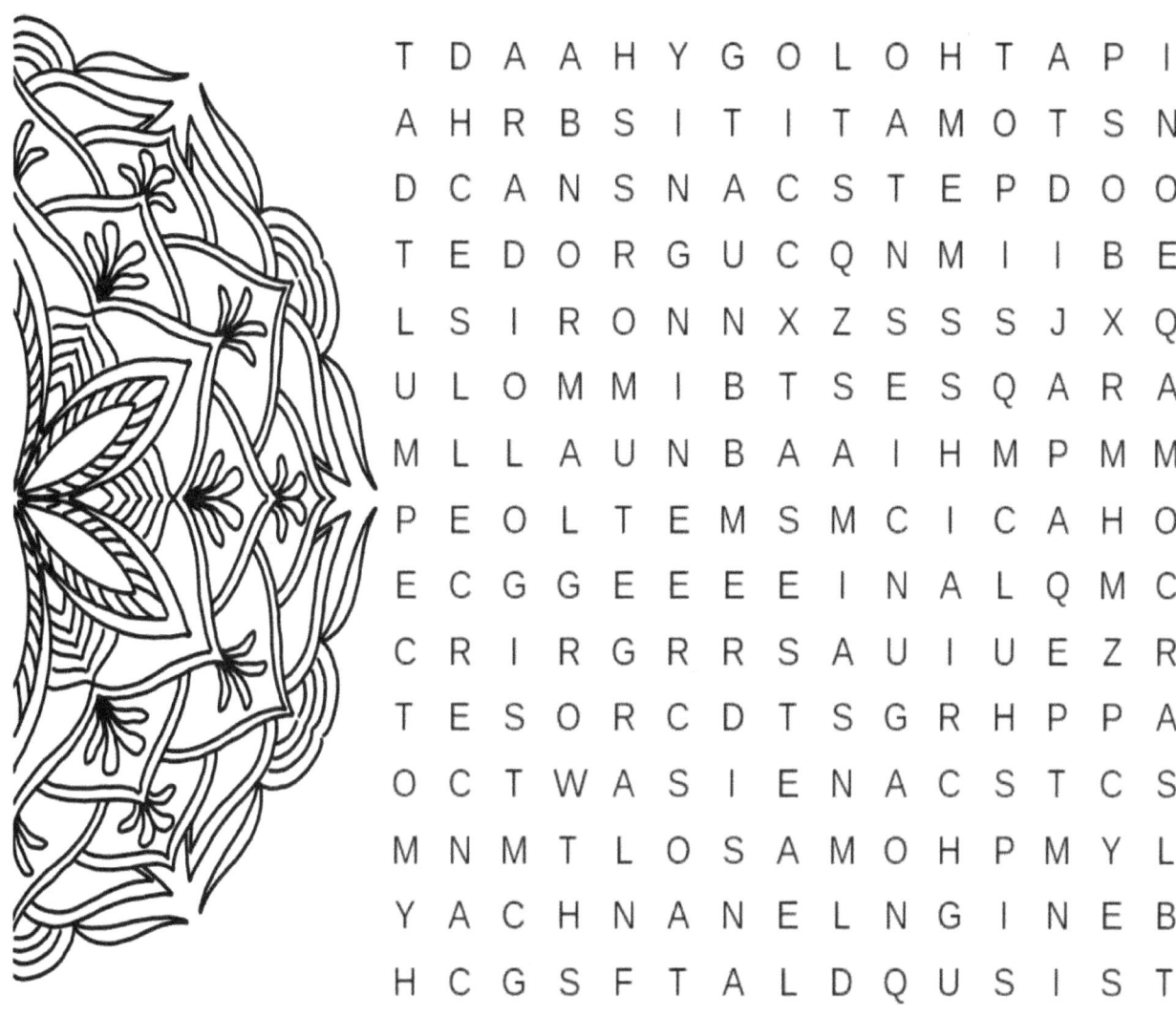

```
T D A A H Y G O L O H T A P I
A H R B S I T I T A M O T S N
D C A N S N A C S T E P D O O
T E D O R G U C Q N M I I B E
L S I R O N N X Z S S S J X Q
U L O M M I B T S E S Q A R A
M L L A U N B A A I H M P M M
P E O L T E M S M C I C A H O
E C G G E E E E I N A L Q M C
C R I R G R R S A U I U E Z R
T E S O R C D T S G R H P P A
O C T W A S I E N A C S T C S
M N M T L O S A M O H P M Y L
Y A C H N A N E L N G I N E B
H C G S F T A L D Q U S I S T
```

WORD LIST:

MASS	EXAMINATION	LUMPECTOMY	RADIOLOGIST
SCREENING	ABNORMAL GROWTHS	LARGE TUMOR	CT SCAN
CAUSES	DISEASE	SARCOMA	PET SCAN
BENIGN	REMISSION	STOMATITIS	MALIGNANT
LYMPHOMAS	PATHOLOGY	CANCER CELLS	CHEMO

© We Survived Publishing

How Are You Feeling Today?

MENTAL HEALTH **PHYSICAL HEALTH**

positive	exhausted	healthy	ill
great	helpless	active	in pain
accomplished	hopeless	energetic	weight gain
frustrated	guilty	fatigued	weight loss
isolated	bothersome	hungry	thirsty
depressed	loveless	no appetite	nauseous
discouraged	ugly	insomnia	bloated
lonely	bored	achy	blockage

Notes: _____

_____

_____

_____

_____

_____

_____

_____

_____

_____

_____

_____

_____

COLON CANCER

(Unscramble these letters to form a word relating to Colon Cancer)

ANSWERS ON PAGE 83

NCOLO _____

CCEARN _____

ECOLACORTL _____

HYEAHTROCMEP _____

OSTOLYMIE _____

ISB _____

ITCLOSI _____

OSYTCOLMO _____

OTMSA BGA _____

WUDON RNEUS _____

PIAN _____

REPDOISSNE _____

AZHIAONIOPSITLT _____

OCLYOOGN _____

DRNTAAIIO _____

KOSBO _____

© We Survived Publishing

How Are You Feeling Today?

MENTAL HEALTH   **PHYSICAL HEALTH**

positive	exhausted	healthy	ill
great	helpless	active	in pain
accomplished	hopeless	energetic	weight gain
frustrated	guilty	fatigued	weight loss
isolated	bothersome	hungry	thirsty
depressed	loveless	no appetite	nauseous
discouraged	ugly	insomnia	bloated
lonely	bored	achy	blockage

Notes: _____

_____

_____

_____

_____

_____

_____

_____

_____

_____

_____

_____

_____

COLON CANCER *SOLVED*

```
A I C A R E G I V E R E D X G R S N D L
N Q S Y E L O S T O M Y S U R V I V O R
E X U Z U Y A H U Y M O T S O E L I G Z
P T N E M E G A N A M N I A P S S R W C
G Z H G A B A M O T S O O J E F E O E O
W E M I S T R W V H Y D M R J C W M G L
O R R X B T W E O I V P E E N B R O E O
U A H M B D O L C J Y A H A G J U S Y R
N C C N H I L M D N Y I C A S A A E T E
D F X Z O I S I A G A N M S Q E K Y R C
N L E Y S I N W O R O C E O S D M A O T
U E X T T P T L E L E N L I O O F S E A
R S E D C I O A O P E V D E T R I L A L
S R R U A C S C X R Y S E S W T H A I I
E B C N V U E A A N T O R I O P T W L L
P N I O H W S W B H L L D L S J B I A C
E I S W O O A W O O O E O O S A M P D B
E R E S P W Z R Q C I C R H O G L S M P
L W D I E T C M U T C E R F I L L O P M
S I N S P I R A T I O N Z E A D B H N K
```

WORD LIST:

- ~~COLON CANCER~~
- ~~PAIN~~
- ~~COLORECTAL~~
- ~~PAIN MANAGEMENT~~
- ~~HOSPITAL~~
- ~~ONCOLOGY~~
- ~~WOUND NURSE~~
- ~~IBD~~
- ~~SLEEP~~
- ~~AWARENESS~~
- ~~STOMA BAG~~
- ~~OSTOMY SURVIVOR~~
- ~~OBESITY~~
- ~~INSPIRATION~~
- ~~HOPE~~
- ~~CHEMO~~
- ~~CAREGIVER~~
- ~~ILEOSTOMY~~
- ~~COLOSTOMY~~
- ~~RECTUM~~
- ~~BOWEL CANCER~~
- ~~CROHNS DISEASE~~
- ~~COLITIS~~
- ~~BATHROOM~~
- ~~STOMA REVERSAL~~
- ~~BLOOD TYPE~~
- ~~LEAKAGE~~
- ~~HOLLISTER~~
- ~~RELAXATION~~
- ~~SELF CARE~~
- ~~DIET~~
- ~~EXERCISE~~

© We Survived Publishing

How Are You Feeling Today?

MENTAL HEALTH **PHYSICAL HEALTH**

positive	exhausted	healthy	ill
great	helpless	active	in pain
accomplished	hopeless	energetic	weight gain
frustrated	guilty	fatigued	weight loss
isolated	bothersome	hungry	thirsty
depressed	loveless	no appetite	nauseous
discouraged	ugly	insomnia	bloated
lonely	bored	achy	blockage

Notes: _____

_____

_____

_____

_____

_____

_____

_____

_____

_____

_____

_____

_____

_____

CANCER SCRAMBLE #1 SOLVED

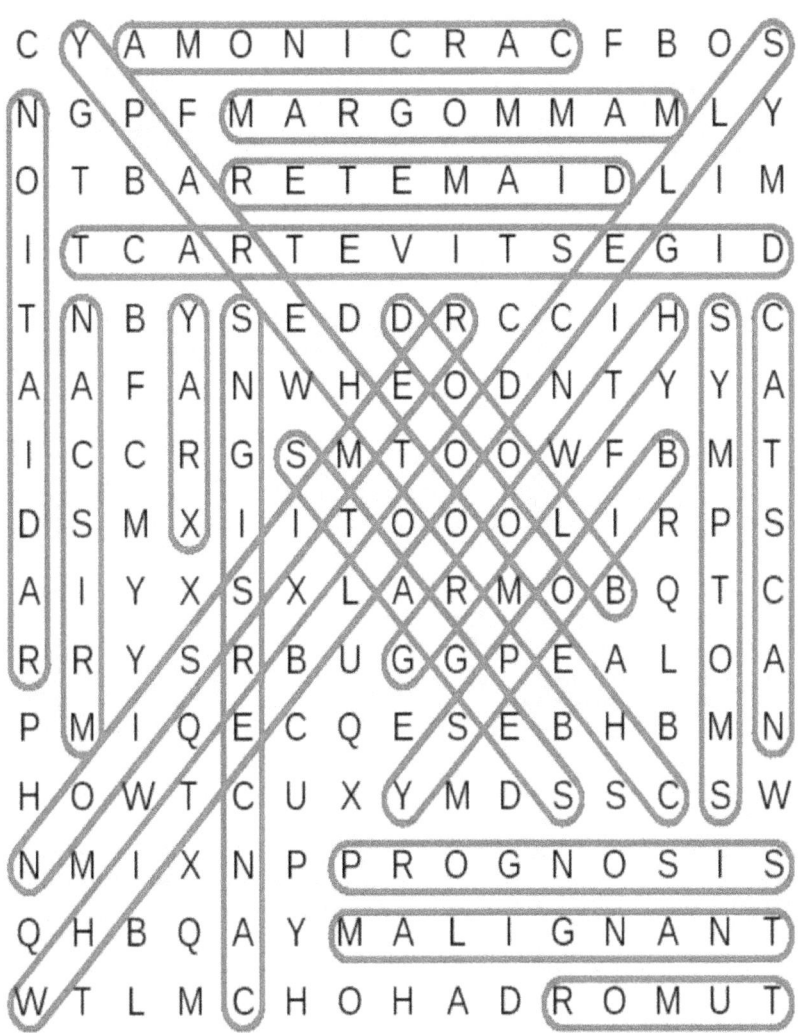

© We Survived Publishing

WORD LIST:

- BLOOD
- CARCINOMA
- CAT SCAN
- MALIGNANT
- MAMMOGRAM
- MRI SCAN
- PROGNOSIS
- XRAY
- CHEMOTHERAPY
- RADIATION
- TUMOR
- WHITEBLOOD CELLS
- REMISSION
- DIAMETER
- STAGES
- DIGESTIVE TRACT
- GROWTH
- BIOPSY
- CANCER SIGNS
- SYMPTOMS

How Are You Feeling Today?

MENTAL HEALTH **PHYSICAL HEALTH**

	positive		exhausted		healthy		ill
	great		helpless		active		in pain
	accomplished		hopeless		energetic		weight gain
	frustrated		guilty		fatigued		weight loss
	isolated		bothersome		hungry		thirsty
	depressed		loveless		no appetite		nauseous
	discouraged		ugly		insomnia		bloated
	lonely		bored		achy		blockage

Notes: _____

_____

_____

_____

_____

_____

_____

_____

_____

_____

_____

_____

_____

THE BODY

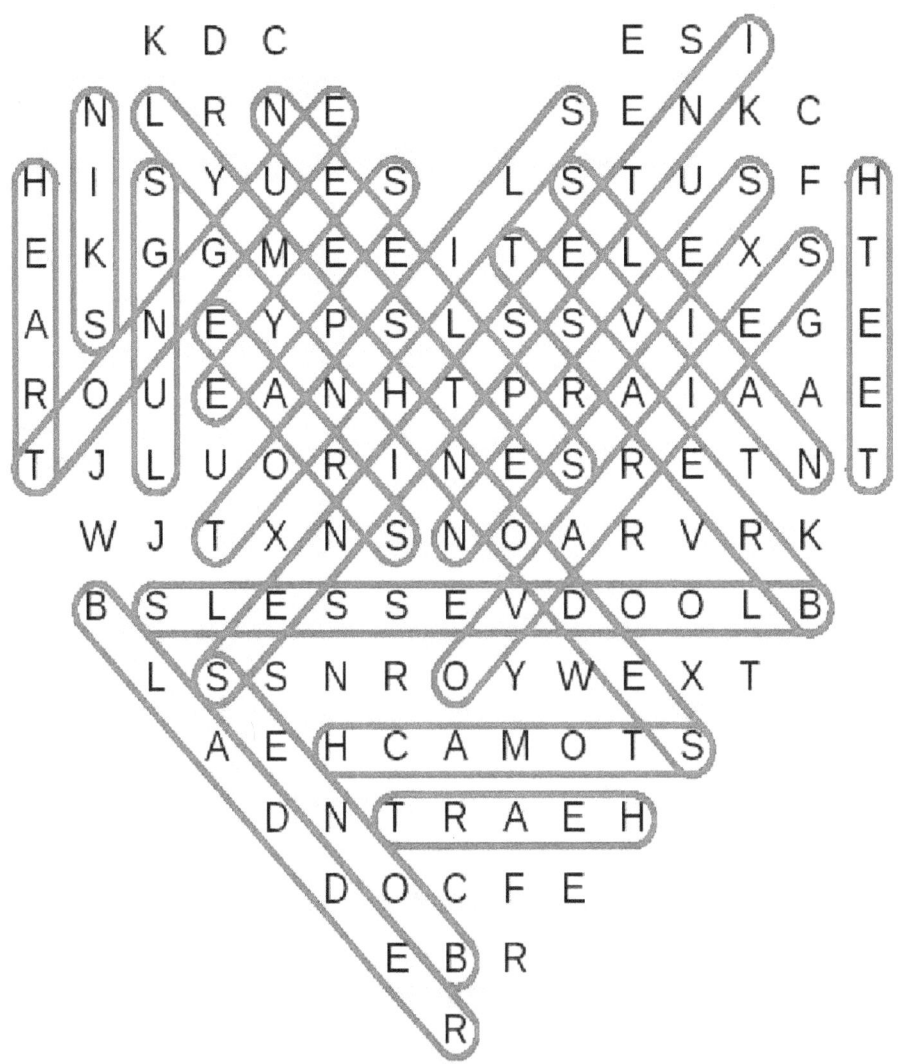

WORD LIST:

SKIN LYMPH NODES TONSILS EYES
NAILS STOMACH LUNGS EARS
BONES INTESTINES HEART HEART
NERVES SPLEEN BLADDER TONGUE
BLOOD VESSELS OVARIES BREAST TEETH

How Are You Feeling Today?

MENTAL HEALTH **PHYSICAL HEALTH**

positive	exhausted	healthy	ill
great	helpless	active	in pain
accomplished	hopeless	energetic	weight gain
frustrated	guilty	fatigued	weight loss
isolated	bothersome	hungry	thirsty
depressed	loveless	no appetite	nauseous
discouraged	ugly	insomnia	bloated
lonely	bored	achy	blockage

Notes: _____

_____

_____

_____

_____

_____

_____

_____

_____

_____

_____

_____

_____

CANCER SCRAMBLE #2   *SOLVED*

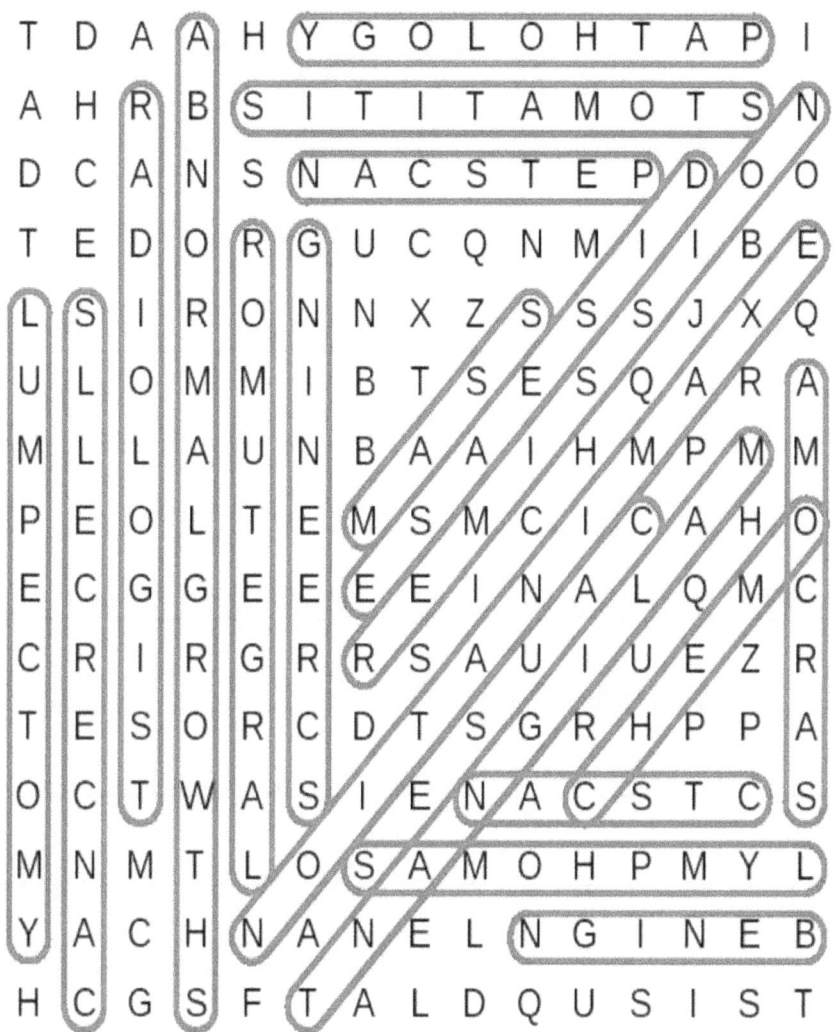

WORD LIST:

- ~~MASS~~
- ~~SCREENING~~
- ~~CAUSES~~
- ~~BENIGN~~
- ~~LYMPHOMAS~~
- ~~EXAMINATION~~
- ~~ABNORMAL GROWTHS~~
- ~~DISEASE~~
- ~~REMISSION~~
- ~~PATHOLOGY~~
- ~~LUMPECTOMY~~
- ~~LARGE TUMOR~~
- ~~SARCOMA~~
- ~~STOMATITIS~~
- ~~CANCER CELLS~~
- ~~RADIOLOGIST~~
- ~~CT SCAN~~
- ~~PET SCAN~~
- ~~MALIGNANT~~
- ~~CHEMO~~

© We Survived Publishing

How Are You Feeling Today?

MENTAL HEALTH　　　　　　　　　**PHYSICAL HEALTH**

	positive		exhausted		healthy		ill
	great		helpless		active		in pain
	accomplished		hopeless		energetic		weight gain
	frustrated		guilty		fatigued		weight loss
	isolated		bothersome		hungry		thirsty
	depressed		loveless		no appetite		nauseous
	discouraged		ugly		insomnia		bloated
	lonely		bored		achy		blockage

Notes: _____

_____

_____

_____

_____

_____

_____

_____

_____

_____

_____

_____

_____

_____

COLON CANCER
(Unscamble Word Answers)

NCOLO	COLON
CCEARN	CANCER
ECOLACORTL	COLORECTAL
HYEAHTROCMEP	CHEMOTHERAPY
OSTOLYMIE	ILEOSTOMY
ISB	IBS
ITCLOSI	COLITIS
OSYTCOLMO	COLOSTOMY
OTMSA BGA	STOMA BAG
WUDON RNEUS	WOUND NURSE
PIAN	PAIN
REPDOISSNE	DEPRESSION
AZHIAONIOPSITLT	HOSPITALIZATION
OCLYOOGN	ONCOLOGY
DRNTAAIIO	RADIATION
KOSBO	BOOKS

© We Survived Publishing

www.ingramcontent.com/pod-product-compliance
Lightning Source LLC
Chambersburg PA
CBHW082019230526
45466CB00022B/2613